If you were offered an extra 15 years of comfortable life without pain or weakness or paralysis or a failing heart, would you take it? If you could look better, feel better, have more pep and a better sex life, would you take the necessary simple steps to achieve these goals?

This book, PREVENTING TYPE 2 DIABETES, will tell you:
- What metabolic syndrome means
- How to recognize the metabolic syndrome
- How to be tested for it
- Why you should start medications as soon as diagnosis is made, *along with* making changes in your lifestyle, *not* waiting months or years for modifications in exercise and diet alone to take effect
- How and why the metabolic syndrome is a family affair, calling for testing and treatment of everyone related to you
- How the metabolic syndrome is linked to type 2 diabetes

You will learn:
- Why fat *in* your belly is more harmful than fat anywhere else and how it differs from the "spare tire" *around* your waist
- How cholesterol and sugar harm your arteries and heart
- Why weight loss helps your body use its own insulin more efficiently
- Why you do not have to become a diabetic, even if you have the genes for diabetes
- Why one or more of your relatives died suddenly at a young age and nobody understood why
- Why metabolic syndrome is often ignored by those who have it
- Why the metabolic syndrome is under-diagnosed and under-treated
- Why the elevated blood sugar is not the most important thing about diabetes
- How and why blood pressure control and cholesterol reduction in the metabolic syndrome can save your life and prevent the onset of type 2 diabetes

Preventing Type 2 Diabetes

Beyond Diet and Exercise

Preventing
Type 2 Diabetes

Beyond Diet and Exercise

Gabriel Hilkovitz, M.B., B.Ch.

BelVista Publishers, LLC
Scottsdale, Arizona

Project Coordinator: Deborah Hilcove
Managing Editor: Patricia Bezunartea
Cover Design: George Foster, Foster Covers
Interior Design: 1106 Design
Figure Credits: Yvonne Smith, VAS Communications
Website Design: Danita Leonard, DL Web Works
Printing: Biltmore ProPrint

Hilkovitz, Gabriel.
        Preventing type 2 diabetes : beyond diet and exercise
        / Gabriel Hilkovitz.
        p. cm.
        Includes bibliographical references and index.
        LCCN 2007933027
        ISBN-13: 978-0-9787080-0-9
        ISBN-10: 0-9787080-0-8

        1. Non-insulin-dependent diabetes--Prevention.
        2. Metabolic syndrome--Treatment.   I. Title.

        RC662.18.H55 2008   616.4'6205
                                         QBI08-600081

BelVista books are available at quantity discounts for corporate training programs, fundraising, or educational endeavors. Custom editions and excerpts can be produced to specification. For more information, contact BelVista Publishers, LLC, PO Box 2723, Scottsdale, AZ 85252-2723 or visit the website, *www.belvistapublishers.com*.

DEDICATION

This book is dedicated to those who struggle daily
with the ravages of diabetes and to their families and caregivers
who work diligently for their well-being.

I hope that the preventive measures outlined
in this book will one day help millions avoid the disease
and its life-threatening complications.

This book is also dedicated to those,
who through their generosity and their social awareness,
will make prevention a reality.

ACKNOWLEDGMENTS

A book such as this is, of course, a synthesis of knowledge and experience gained over many years. Some is self-taught, but most of it derives from the writings, teachings and experiments of others who make astute clinical observations or allow their genius to work in laboratories behind the scenes.

I am grateful to the professors who instructed me as a student, intern and resident in South Africa, England and America. I have also learned from nurses, patients, laboratory technicians, and from other doctors. I owe a debt of gratitude to them all.

Special thanks are owed to my wife, Deborah, and our dear friend, Patricia Bezunartea, for supervising this project. I appreciate my son, Michael, who has understood the importance of this book. Lloyd and Amanda Brenden, Malcolm and Peggy Hilcove, Bill and Cheri Lay, and Sarah Hilkovitz Smith have offered insights, support and encouragement.

I have come also to appreciate how many people help produce a book. I owe special thanks to George Foster for his fine cover design and his friendship; to Michele DeFilippo of 1106 Design for the interior design; to Yvonne Smith of VAS Communications for interpreting my sketches into illustrations; to Danita Leonard of DL Web Works for the website design; to Jeff Adler of Quiesco for keeping the computers up and running; to Phil and Aaron Quartullo of Biltmore ProPrint for printing the book and helping to meet deadlines; to Jack Harthun, Cheri Craig, Larry Zeller, Mike Mansel, and Lloyd Rich for their professional expertise; to ABPA, PMA and Independent Publishers Group for believing in this book.

From the Arizona Heart Institute, the Arizona Heart Hospital and the Arizona Heart Foundation, my thanks go to Dr. Edward Diethrich, Dr. William Rappoport, Yvonne Smith, Kristin Conant, Amanda Marinelli, Jill Rogers, Nancy Williams-Boyle, Shelley Anonson, Nancy Ashland, Susan Roth and Gerry Kroloff. I've appreciated the AHI and AHH staff members who have been interested in this project and cheered the progress. I owe special thanks to Arlene Michaelson for her quiet efficiency and good humor.

Family, friends and patients have believed in this book and its purpose in preventing type 2 diabetes. Many, many dear people have helped bring about this book, including Rose Amendola, Victor and Flora Arroyo, Jerry and Gena Aslanian, Germain and Betty Ball, Harvey and Eileen Barish, Barbara Bening, Jacqui Berns, Cindy Bezunartea, John and Sherill Boyle, Hilton and Kate Braithwaite, Peter and Janet Casper, James and Dorothy Cameron, Gayle Collins and Barbara Sheen, David and Bonnie Cowan, Ron and Karin Crissey, Winson and Karen DeWitt, Terry and Susan Driescher, Mary Eggstaff, Ted and Rachel Elizondo, David Espinoza, Marcia Fine, Martin and Ellen Friend, Don and Amelia Garrison, John and Maxine Goodson, Jean Gould, Alphonse Granatek, Barbara Granquist, Joe Gulotta, Dave and Amy Harper, Jack and Mary Harthun, Gill Hilcove, Kelly Hilcove, Maurice and Dorothy Hilcove, Stuart Hilcove, Andrea Hilkovitz, Dana Hock, Bruce and Lydia Holmes, Arlene Jacobson, Philip and Barbara Karpouskas, Carole Klein, Stanley and Mary Klock, Ken Lange, Bruce and Jane Lawson, Barry Lay, Susan Lentz, Don and Isabelle Lisa, Bruce Lutz, Virginia McLeod, Kenneth and Josephine McElligott, John and Nadine Maruca, Bill Mast, Gary and Cindy May, Mike and Colleen Manley, Sharon Metzger, Marsha Meyer, Myra Mihotic, Carl and Claire Muecke, William and Marion Nenstiel, Mike and Brenda Nitchen, James and Janie Norman, Dallas Ortman, Adilson Pascui, Katherleen Person, Arthur Plant, Kevin and Glynnis Podmore, Sue Putzier, Virginia Rader, Jack Ralston, Augustin and Bertha Ramirez, William and Tula Rappoport, Lillian Rees, James and Frankie Sampley, Darlene Saunders, Al Schmitt, Jordi Schumann, Frances Scianni, Rachel Sellens, Ralph and Geraldine Sherrill, William and Cheryl Shisler, William and Angela Showalter, Rita Silverman, Chris Sweeney, Mike Sweeney, Carmella Tibshraeny, Sid Tibshraeny, Karen Towle, Richard and Edwina Traylor, Florence Umphrey, Judy Walker, William and JoAnne Walsh, Pamela Waterman, Angela Waters, Sam and Faye Watkins, Edith Watson, Whitney and Genevieve White, Ken and Beverly Wible, George and Mary Wulitich, Joseph and Mali Wynn, Gene and Susan Yadon.

I am indebted to all who have encouraged me in this effort. I also want to thank, in advance, those who read this book and pass along the information to any who might benefit from it. Prevention is possible, and we must do all we can to make it a reality.

TABLE OF CONTENTS

1

THE LOOMING EPIDEMIC

A national tragedy exists: 40 million Americans are diabetic and 60 million more are in danger of developing diabetes. In the United States, more than 200 people die every day from diabetes and its consequences. Recent newspaper reports suggest one American in five is or will become diabetic, and babies born after the year 2000 have a one in three chance of becoming diabetic.

Diabetes and its complications — strokes, blindness, painful neuritis, kidney failure, loss of limbs, heart attacks — are the most expensive diseases to treat, accounting for well over half of Medicare's budget.

Not only is the disease killing us, but it is also crippling our economy and sending health care costs spiraling upward.

However, preventive measures are available, waiting to be used effectively on a national scale.

Americans should be the fittest, not the fattest, nation on earth. We are losing our competitive edge physically and economically. We are weakened by a preventable disease of epidemic proportions and crippled economically by enormous health care expenditures.

This book is about preventing diabetes and about recognizing those who run the risk of becoming diabetics. It describes a stage called pre-diabetes, or the metabolic syndrome, and explains how to detect and manage it.

The media has focused on obesity, and nearly every magazine and newspaper carries information about it. However, obesity is only one facet of the metabolic syndrome. Genetics, race, inactivity, poor food choices, high blood pressure and cholesterol abnormalities are all parts of this condition, affecting nearly 60 million Americans including children and adolescents.

Most importantly, this book explains and ties together each aspect of the pre-diabetic condition, putting complex issues into simple words.

This book can help individuals, their families, their friends and the community prevent type 2 diabetes, saving billions of healthcare dollars and avoiding widespread, severe suffering.

2

DIABETES FROM
MY PERSPECTIVE

After graduating from medical school, followed by internships and residencies in teaching hospitals in South Africa and later in England and America, I frequently saw diabetes. Many hospital admissions were the result of either low blood sugar reactions to insulin, or comas resulting from diabetic keto-acidosis or from very high blood sugars. Whereas a normal nonfasting blood sugar runs about 120 mg, sometimes these blood sugars were over 1000 mg per 100 ml!

Such extremes were common because home glucose monitors were unknown, and insulin dosage was more or less guesswork based on inaccurate urine tests. Before doctors knew how to test urine for glucose, they had to taste the urine for sweetness. Thank goodness those days are gone!

Other fairly common problems included gestational diabetes in pregnancy; difficult deliveries due to large babies born by weakened, diabetic mothers; diabetic or "wet" gangrene in infected toes and feet; and slow-healing traumatic and surgical wounds often complicated by infection in the era before effective antibiotics.

We spoke then of "juvenile" and "adult-onset" diabetes, characterizing them as either insulin-dependent or non-insulin-dependent. These are now known as types 1 and 2.

The association between obesity and type 2 diabetes was evident, but little was known about cholesterol and its intimate connection to vascular disease. Hypertension was treated with salt restriction, weight reduction and sedatives or surgical sympathectomy, which is an operation cutting the sympathetic nerves next to the spinal cord in order to reduce blood pressure.

The common association between cardiovascular disease and diabetes was recognized, but the cause and effect connections were not realized until the 1960s.

Insulin was derived from cows and pigs. Reactions to the foreign animal protein were fairly common, and antibodies to the beef or pork protein sometimes rendered those insulins ineffective.

In type 2 diabetes, insulin was often seen as a "last resort medicine" after oral agents had failed. Patients were sometimes threatened with insulin injections if they did not comply with dietary restrictions and other treatments. Little was known then about beta cell fatigue and the specific indications for the early use of insulin to prevent beta cell exhaustion.

Such difficulties and lack of knowledge affected my experiences with diabetic patients and led to frustration.

In England, I was responsible for running an out-patient diabetic program in a teaching hospital. There were no glucose monitors, and patients attended the clinic about once a month to have urine tested or to have fasting blood sugars drawn. Some patients fasted longer than required to impress the doctors with their low blood sugar.

Dietary prescriptions were based on complex "exchange lists" which the majority of patients did not understand. In post-war England, even in the 1950s, proteins were expensive, whereas starches were the mainstay of many diets. In spite of these deficiencies, I am certain that many diabetics benefited from the lack of automobiles and expensive "petrol" because they had to walk everywhere. Additionally, many were avid gardeners which provided them some exercise as well as abundant vegetables.

When the longer-acting, human insulins became available and glucose monitors were used more frequently, the overall picture improved considerably.

A little historical perceptive leads to the realization that we are indeed fortunate today in our better understanding of cholesterol abnormalities and hypertension and their role in diabetes. Better insulins and recently discovered medications offer a multi-dimensional approach to treatment and glucose control. With recognition of the metabolic syndrome and the pre-diabetic insulin resistant state, type 2 diabetes can be prevented.

However, even if stem-cell and other research allows us to transplant or regenerate new pancreatic beta cells, the fundamental challenges of obesity and insulin resistance, of cholesterol abnormalities and hypertension will be with us for decades to come. These metabolic precursors of diabetes will cause new beta cells to fail again and create yet another generation of diabetics.

Diabetes will kill thousands of Americans this year. It will require health care expenditures exceeding $115 billion annually in this country alone. It will cost lost wages and lost company profits. It will result in blindness, kidney failure, dialysis, and death. It will leave orphans, widowers and widows.

Even though tremendous advancements have been made in treating this horrible disease, it is heart-wrenching that millions of patients and caregivers are unaware of new prevention and treatment options and are thereby prolonging the ravages of diabetes.

Prevention is possible, and it is imperative to educate patients and their families.

3

OVERVIEW OF THE METABOLIC SYNDROME

The Link between Metabolic Syndrome and Type 2 Diabetes

Metabolic syndrome is often pre-diabetes. Early detection and treatment of the metabolic syndrome can:

- Prevent type 2 diabetes
- Reduce heart attacks and strokes
- Help make you insurable
- Reduce your medical bills
- Save you from blindness
- Preserve your kidneys
- Prevent amputations
- Add 10–20 years to your life

> ## Is This You?
>
> - Overweight
> - Big waistline (over 35" for women, and over 40" for men)
> - Elevated blood pressure
> - Abnormal cholesterol and triglycerides
> - Family history of diabetes
>
> **If you answer "Yes" to any three of these conditions, you have the metabolic syndrome and your life is in danger!**

■ Some Alarming Statistics

Diabetes is responsible for more cases of heart disease and kidney failure than any other disease. Nearly one out of five Americans has diabetes or is at high risk for developing it.

The annual cost of treating diabetes and its complications in the United States exceeds $115 billion.

Every single day in the United States, diabetes is the cause of at least:

- 200 deaths (80% of diabetics die from vascular and heart problems)
- 150 amputations
- 70 cases of blindness (diabetic retinal disease is the leading cause of blindness in persons between the ages of 20 and 65)
- 55 cases of kidney failure
- and hundreds of heart attacks and strokes (the risk of a heart attack is 2–4 times higher in a diabetic).

In the United States alone:
- 60 million people have pre-diabetes and 5% of those are children
- an additional 15 million people are unaware that they have diabetes
- 40 million people have diabetes

These are alarming statistics! Yet, this does not have to be the case. We can decrease the incidence of diabetes if we learn to recognize the symptoms of pre-diabetes or metabolic syndrome early and immediately begin a vigorous campaign to keep the metabolic syndrome from developing into type 2 diabetes.

■ The Case for Prevention

EARLY RECOGNITION

> By the time diabetes is diagnosed, most patients already have significant heart disease. This implies that cardiovascular disease begins in the pre-diabetic, insulin resistant stage called the metabolic syndrome.
> **Early recognition of metabolic syndrome can prevent type 2 diabetes**

Many people believe diabetes is mainly a disease of high blood sugar and good control of their sugar is all that is needed to avoid problems. They know there is a connection between being overweight and having diabetes. There has been a lot of publicity about the increase of obesity — even among teenagers and young children — and the rising incidence of diabetes.

However, most do not understand the connection between obesity, the metabolic syndrome and the resulting complications of type 2 diabetes. They do not understand the relationship between sugar — or glucose — and the devastating results of diabetes.

DIABETES IS DEADLY

> **The reason to be concerned is that metabolic syndrome, like diabetes, can kill.**
> **Both can shorten life. Both create painful suffering and serious disabilities.**
> **Both affect an entire family.**

Obesity and the associated metabolic syndrome are on the rise, even attacking teenagers in epidemic proportions. The incidence of diabetes doubled in the 1990s. The causes for this are well known: lack of exercise and physical activities, coupled with poor eating habits emphasizing fatty, processed and carbohydrate-laden foods, washed down with sugary drinks.

DIABETES IS COSTLY

Metabolic syndrome leads to diabetes and cardiovascular disease. Diabetics are heavy consumers of medical care, and diabetes is one of the costliest diseases to treat. Diabetics with kidney failure account for the highest proportion of dialysis patients. In addition, diabetics also account for the highest proportion of patients requiring cardiovascular intervention, such as by-pass surgery, angioplasties and stents.

UNDER-UTILIZED PREVENTION AND TREATMENT

Today, we understand better how glucose, a relatively inert chemical, can harm blood vessels. We have also shifted from overemphasizing glucose control toward treating the inflammation in blood vessels. This is done by 1) more aggressively lowering blood pressure and cholesterol to new and healthier target levels and 2) treating insulin resistance.

At present, both prevention and treatment are under-utilized. Few patients with diabetes know their cholesterol is elevated. Even fewer diabetics are being treated for high cholesterol, and among those, only a very small percentage has reached ideal cholesterol levels. Similarly, elevated blood pressure remains an under-treated problem.

Professional and lay publications reflect some of these changes in emphasis from glucose control toward treating the inflammation of blood vessels. However, the message is not getting through to patients, their families, their doctors and other caregivers.

One reason for this is the fatalistic and incorrect notion that diabetes is purely a genetic disease. Many diabetics and their families believe current treatments are merely "band-aids" and one day there will be a momentous breakthrough to cure diabetes.

Another reason may be the lack of understanding and knowledge about new treatments and the extent to which they can make the outlook more optimistic if these treatments are started early.

EARLY DIAGNOSIS AND TREATMENT OF METABOLIC SYNDROME CAN *PREVENT* TYPE 2 DIABETES

Do *not* wait until your blood sugar becomes elevated before starting a prevention program. **Metabolic syndrome can be identified as much as 10 to 15 years before type 2 diabetes occurs.** During that window of time, the cardiovascular complications of metabolic syndrome can be identified and reversed through proper medications and lifestyle changes *(Fig. 1)*.

Regardless of age, sex or race, everyone who has a large waistline — central obesity — should be tested for metabolic syndrome, also known as pre-diabetes.

Doctors and other caregivers should impress upon people with pre-diabetes that treatment, using medications to control obesity, high blood pressure and cholesterol abnormalities, is of the greatest urgency and importance. **Treatment should achieve the recommended targets for blood pressure and cholesterol correction over a short period of time (3 months).** Weight loss is a slow process but even a 10 pound weight loss can be achieved within 3 months.

Evolution of Diabetes

Overworked pancreatic beta cells in the metabolic syndrome become fatigued, producing insufficient insulin in diabetes.

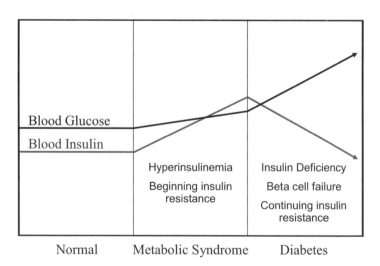

Figure 1

4

FEATURES OF THE
METABOLIC SYNDROME

A wareness and recognition of the markers of metabolic syndrome is an important step in the prevention of type 2 diabetes.

- Central Obesity — waist measurement over 35" for women, and 40" for men.
- Body Mass Index (BMI) over 25
- High Triglycerides — over 150 mg/dl
- High Fasting Glucose — over 100 mg/dl
- Low HDL-C — Less than 45 mg/dl of High Density Lipoprotein, the "good" cholesterol
- High Blood Pressure — over 130/80 mmHg

■ Central Obesity: The Enemy Within Us

Nearly every magazine, newspaper and television report has focused on the problem of obesity. However, some types of fat are more harmful than others. For the purpose of this book, there are two major groups.

TWO TYPES OF BODY FAT: "PEARS AND APPLES"

Fat on lower parts of the body, such as the hips and buttocks, gives the "pear-shaped" body appearance. This fat is storage fat. It does not behave like the fat within the abdomen, but it is evidence, of course, that the individual has been eating far more than necessary, and the body has stored excess energy as fat.

However, fat *within* the abdomen, packed around the intestines and other internal organs, is a major cause of heart and arterial disease, both in the metabolic syndrome and in diabetes. Central obesity is characteristic of the "apple-shaped" body and contributes to the big waist measurement.

Fat cells *in* the abdomen behave differently from fat cells *on* the abdomen — those which are sometimes called a "spare tire" — and they are far more dangerous. The abdominal fat cells in obese persons do not release enough adiponectin, a hormone which protects the blood vessels.

Also, the fat cells inside the abdomen are constantly releasing fatty acids into the blood going to the liver. Some of these fatty acids are first converted into triglycerides and then into the lipoproteins VLDL-C, IDL-C and LDL-C, described in the Terminology chapter under "Cholesterol" and "Triglycerides."

The fat inside the abdomen contains immune cells called "macrophages," which release inflammatory hormones and chemical compounds harmful to blood vessels, including interleukin-6 and tumor necrosis factor alpha (IL-6 and TNF-alpha).

Furthermore, these fat cells in the abdomen release a hormone called "resistin," causing insulin resistance. Some fatty acids reach the muscles where they contribute to insulin resistance. This is the inability of muscle cells to use insulin properly either to burn glucose or store it as glycogen.

There is a class of medications to help with this problem. "Fibrates" are medications that slow the breakdown of fat cells within the abdomen. Therefore, they reduce the amount of fatty acids going to the liver. This reduction, in turn, decreases the formation of triglycerides and LDL-C. The liver, now less preoccupied with processing fatty acids, can produce more of the *good* cholesterol HDL-C.

Abdominal obesity is a better predictor of coronary heart disease than body mass index (BMI). People with the largest waist measurements run a risk of heart disease 9 times greater than those with smaller waists. Women should strive for waist measurements no more than 35 inches, while men should aim for no more than 40 inches.

■ Body Mass Index (BMI)

Maintaining a BMI in the normal range helps eliminate obesity as a risk factor for coronary artery disease and for metabolic syndrome and type 2 diabetes.

BMI relates weight to body surface area. For example, a BMI of 25 means you weigh 25 kilograms per square meter of body surface area.

A BMI over 25 means you are overweight

A BMI over 30 means you are obese *(see Fig. 2)*

■ Triglycerides should be less than 150 mg/dl

Triglycerides are absorbed from the food and packaged into chylomicrons which then travel to the liver for processing. Triglycerides become part of the cholesterol molecules. This is explained more fully in the chapter about treating cholesterol abnormalities.

■ Fasting blood sugar level

After fasting 8 hours, your blood sugar should be 100mg/dl or less if you do not have the metabolic syndrome *(Fig. 3)*.

If your fasting blood sugar is between 100 and 120 mg/dl you have "impaired fasting glucose" (IFG), a marker for metabolic syndrome.

If your fasting blood sugar is over 120 mg/dl, you have diabetes.

Blood sugar can also be measured 2 hours after a meal or 2 hours after a dose of 75G of glucose. Normally, the blood sugar should not exceed 140 mg/dl. *(Fig. 3)*

Body Mass Index (BMI)

BMI = Weight in kilograms per
square meter of body surface area

Height - no shoes (feet, inches)	Ideal Weight in Pounds BMI of 24-25
4'10"	110-115
4'11"	115-120
5'0"	120-125
5'1"	125-130
5'2"	130-135
5'3"	135-140
5'4"	140-145
5'5"	145-150
5'6"	150-155
5'7"	155-160
5'8"	160-165
5'9"	165-170
5'10"	170-175
5'11"	175-180
6'0"	180-185
6'1"	185-190
6'2"	190-195
6'3"	195-200
6'4"	200-205

Figure 2

If it is more than 140 mg/100 ml, you have "impaired glucose tolerance" (IGT), a marker for metabolic syndrome.

Many physicians now believe a blood sugar of 160 mg/dl or more, after a meal, indicates diabetes.

■ Low HDL-C (less than 45 mg/dl) is a strong predictor of heart disease

HDL-C The *"good"* cholesterol should be over 45 mg/dl in males and over 50 mg/dl in females

LDL-C The *"bad"* cholesterol should be 70 mg/dl or less.

The LDL-C (the "bad" cholesterol, also known as low-density lipoprotein) is usually not elevated in the metabolic syndrome, but it exists as small particles which are more likely to set up plaque formation.

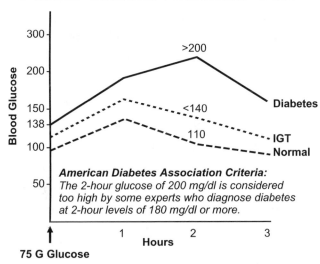

3-Hour Glucose Tolerance Test

IGT - Impaired Glucose Tolerance
2 hour blood glucose <200 mg/dl
Diabetes - 2 hour blood glucose
>200 mg/dl

- Normal fasting blood glucose < 100 mg/dl
- Impaired glucose tolerance fasting blood glucose <125 mg/dl
  Metabolic Syndrome (insulin resistance)
- Diabetes Fasting blood glucose >125 mg/dl

Figure 3

Particle size can now be measured in advanced cholesterol tests which are becoming standard practice. These tests are covered by many insurance plans.

Raising HDL-C using niacin, statins, or fibrates reduces heart disease significantly. Exercise and diet are far less effective in raising HDL-C than medication. This is a strong argument for not relying on lifestyle changes alone to reduce the risk of a heart attack in a pre-diabetic or in a patient with type 2 diabetes.

■ Blood pressure should be 130/80 mmHg (mercury) or less to be normal

The top number is the systolic pressure measured in the arm over the brachial artery just after the heart has pumped. The bottom reading is the diastolic pressure recorded when the heart is relaxed between pumps.

The blood pressure cuff is connected to a mercury column which shows the pressure in millimeters of mercury (mmHg).

Blood pressure fluctuates with rest, activity, stress, anger, sleep and daily living. The "normal" blood pressure refers to the reading when a person is relaxed and calm. The blood pressure may be higher in the doctor's office, due perhaps to anxiety. This is so common that it is referred to as "white coat syndrome." Blood pressure may be lower at home, in calm and familiar surroundings.

Even when the blood pressure is "normal," it may fluctuate by 5 to 10 mmHg. By definition, an elevated blood pressure is one that remains high even when the person is relaxed and calm.

The blood pressure should be the same or similar in both arms.

> **Prevention is up to you.**
> **No one else can do it for you.**
> **Early detection and treatment of metabolic**
> **syndrome can save your life!**

Knowledge Can Save Your Life

"Every day brings a new challenge when you're caring for someone with diabetes," she told me during the office visit with her diabetic husband, a new patient.

Her husband, barely 48, had already had one heart attack and had lost most of the vision in one eye. Now, a deep ulcer had developed on the sole of one foot where he used to have a callous.

"We were so careful with his diet after we learned he had diabetes, and we followed instructions about his feet, too," she sighed.

"Do you test his blood sugars?" I asked.

"Yes," she answered, "Every morning and every night at bedtime."

It was my turn to sigh. "Didn't your doctor teach you to test two hours after each meal?" I asked.

When she said "No," I answered, "So those blood sugar tests you thought were normal had no connection with his meals?"

"I guess," she replied. "Nobody ever mentioned testing after meals."

I explained that by testing before *meals, he was missing the high blood sugars that occur after eating when foods — especially the carbohydrates or starches — are absorbed from the bowel and cause elevated blood sugars.*

Pre-meal testing often gives a false impression that the blood sugar is normal or near-normal. Diabetics who test their blood sugar first thing in the morning, before eating anything, are getting the best reading of the day, but they may be fooling themselves into thinking their results show they can eat "anything."

That's why I need a measurement two hours after *you begin eating so we can measure how the insulin in your body is handling — or not handling — the sugar or glucose. Remember, now, that "sugar" or glucose in the blood comes from carbohydrates in the food. That's why you have to be careful about what you are eating as well as the quantity of your food. And it's important to eat at fairly regular times every day — and don't skip breakfast.*

I maintained the same medications, trying not to change too many things so we could figure out how his body was using the insulin. I showed him how to keep daily sugar charts and asked him to be sure to bring them to each office visit. Then at future visits, I would be able to adjust his medications according to the test results and sugar charts.

I also referred him to a wound clinic.

They returned after 10 days with his sugar chart in hand. This showed that after meals, his blood sugar was well above 250 mg/dl most of the time. The way they had been testing, first thing in the morning before breakfast, his blood sugar was usually around 120 mg/dl. At bedtime, about 5 hours after the evening meal, it was around 140 mg/dl.

"What you're seeing now is that the blood sugar reaches high peaks 2 hours after his meals, and his medicine has not been controlling those highs," I explained.

"That's why the long term blood sugar test I ran at his first visit was 8%, when it should have been 6%," I emphasized. "Those high sugar peaks do the most damage to the eyes and the kidneys. In reality, the damage to his eyes began a long time ago, before you knew he had diabetes."

Noting her puzzled look, I explained, "Before people become diabetic, they go through a stage called pre-diabetes, when they have resistance to their own insulin and have only mildly elevated blood sugars. In that stage, they have high cholesterol numbers and develop severe disease in the coronary arteries. That's why he had a heart attack — not from high blood sugar — but from high blood fats called triglycerides and a type of low-density lipoprotein, or LDL, which is particularly harmful to the arteries because of the small particle size. And, he probably had high blood pressure, too," I guessed.

"Oh, yes," she said. "But he didn't take his medicine for blood pressure regularly, because they said it wasn't too high, and he could bring it down with exercise and losing weight."

"Did you do those things?" I asked my new patient.

"No," he replied, adding, "At first I lost about 5 pounds, but then my weight went up and down, and I just gave up."

His wife added, "I didn't really understand the diet — counting calories was hard for us. Counting carbs is a lot easier. I never understood how good choices of food can make you feel better."

I wish that I had known them 10 years before his heart attack. I believe I could have encouraged him to exercise, maybe just by walking around the block or parking the car further from the store or using the stairs instead of an elevator or escalator.

I could have shown her how much easier it is to control a diet by watching carbohydrates, not counting calories. And I know I could have attacked the cholesterol problems with medication and treated his blood pressure aggressively.

I would have shown them that type 2 diabetes could be prevented with tests and appropriate medication, beyond diet and exercise.

5
TERMINOLOGY

Before proceeding further with the discussion of the metabolic syndrome and its relation to type 2 diabetes, it is important to understand some words and terms used in this book. The glossary at the back of this book provides a more complete listing of terms.

INSULIN is a hormone made by beta cells in the pancreas. Insulin acts by helping glucose (sugar) enter cells where glucose is needed for energy. Insulin also has important functions in fat and protein metabolism.

INSULIN RESISTANCE is an important factor in both the metabolic syndrome and in type 2 diabetes. It accounts for failure to handle glucose efficiently, but it is also the underlying reason for abnormalities in fat and protein metabolism.

HYPERTENSION means high blood pressure — not nervous tension. The top reading (systolic pressure) is the pressure in the artery just after the heart has pumped. The bottom reading (diastolic pressure) is the pressure in the artery when the heart is relaxed between pumps. The pressure is measured in millimeters of mercury, written mmHg.

The normal blood pressure in the arm (brachial artery) is 100 to 130 systolic and 60 to 80 diastolic.

| Normal Blood Pressure | $\underline{100 \to 130}$ | Systolic |
| in mmHG | $60 \to 80$ | Diastolic |

CHOLESTEROL is an important and normal part of hormones and cell walls. It is a waxy substance that must be combined with protein in order to dissolve in the fluid part of the blood.

Only a small amount of cholesterol comes from food. Most of it is made by the liver, which secretes some of it in the bile which goes to the intestine to assist digestion. Cholesterol is re-absorbed from the intestine and recycled into bile. Some cholesterol enters the blood stream to be carried to parts of the body that need it to make hormones and cell membranes.

- **Cholesterol was named for its presence in bile**
  Chole = Bile   Sterol = A solid alcohol
- **Cholesterol + Protein = Lipoprotein**
      The protein part of cholesterol is called APO lipoprotein. It keeps cholesterol in solution and allows cholesterol to react with other substances in the blood.
- **Lipoproteins are classified according to their density**
      LDL is low density lipoprotein
      HDL is high density lipoprotein
      VLDL is very low density lipoprotein
- All of the lipoproteins contain cholesterol, so we write them to show their cholesterol content as follows:
                LDL-C is 50% cholesterol
                HDL-C is 20% cholesterol
                VLDL-C is 12% cholesterol

TRIGLYCERIDE is a fatty substance made by the liver. Fat in food is digested down into fatty acids and glycerol. These substances are repackaged by the intestinal wall into small particles called "chylomicrons" which are 95% triglyceride and less than 5% cholesterol.

- Chylomicrons enter the intestinal lymphatic vessels, then the veins above the heart, and are carried to the liver.
- The liver also manufactures triglycerides from sugar and starches.
- Trigylceride leaves the liver as VLDL-C, which is 60% triglyceride, 12% cholesterol. Compare this with the LDL-C which is 10% triglyceride, 50% cholesterol, and with the HDL-C which is 5% triglyceride, 20% cholesterol.

HDL-C is the *good* cholesterol because its APO proteins pick up the unused cholesterol and carry it back to the liver. It can be thought of as the "garbage collector."

Triglyceride leaves the liver as VLDL-C which is changed to IDL-C (intermediate density lipoprotein), which is changed to LDL-C. The triglyceride content goes down, whereas the cholesterol content goes up when you go from VLDL-C to IDL-C to LDL-C.

LDL-C is the *"bad cholesterol."* It penetrates the arterial lining and forms part of the harmful plaque. LDL-C is more harmful if it exists as small particles. There are special tests available now to measure particle size and, importantly, there are medications to change small particles into less harmful large particles.

IN THE METABOLIC SYNDROME

- Triglycerides are high > 150 mg/dl
- HDL-C is too low < 45 mg/dl
- LDL-C is normal in amount but the particles are mainly small and more harmful

GOALS OF CHOLESTEROL MANAGEMENT
- Reduce triglycerides below 150 mg/dl
- Raise HDL-C above 50 mg/dl
- Change LDL-C from small to large particles
- Reduce LDL-C below 100 mg/dl using medications such as statins and TZDs

ENDOTHELIUM is the thin, glossy lining of blood vessels.

A healthy endothelium allows blood cells and cholesterol particles to flow easily over it. An unhealthy endothelium, however, becomes sticky and rough, so cells stick to it, forming clots.

LDL-C burrows through the endothelium to start plaque formation. The plaques can swell into the channels where blood flows (the lumen) or the plaques can build up undetected in the wall of the vessels and then rupture like volcanoes, spewing cholesterol and other material into the lumen, suddenly and totally blocking the artery *(Fig. 4)*.

This is what causes heart attacks and strokes — the sudden rupture of those little "volcanoes."

By contrast, the plaques that build up slowly, gradually closing off blood flow, give warning of their existence. These warning symptoms include pain in the heart muscle or angina, when a coronary artery is closing up, or leg cramps in the calf muscles (known as claudication), when you walk, meaning that the arteries of the legs are getting narrow. These slow-growing, artery-narrowing plaques are the ones that are treated with balloons (or angioplasty), and stents.

The vulnerable "volcanoes" rupture without warning. We do not even know they are there unless special ultrasound imaging of the arteries is done. It is correct to assume that everyone with metabolic syndrome already has vulnerable plaques *(Fig. 4)*.

Vulnerable Plaque, Plaque Rupture and Action of Statins

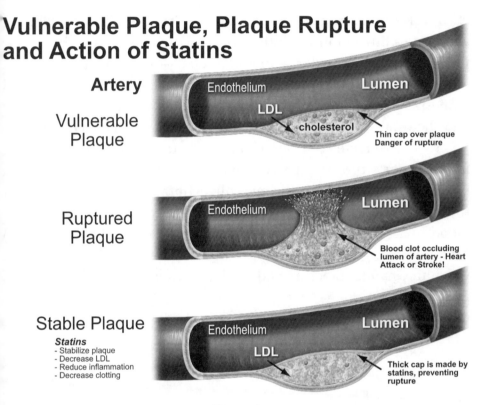

Figure 4

One of the main arguments for starting anti-cholesterol and anti-plaque medicines early is to halt plaque formation and to strengthen the caps over potential volcanoes so they will not rupture.

Exercise and diet alone will NOT do this, but the statin medications will. You cannot rely on exercise and diet to prevent the rupture of these vulnerable plaques.

ENDOTHELIAL INFLAMMATION is the burrowing of small LDL-C particles under the endothelium, and then the infiltration of the vessel wall by certain cells that release super oxides and other chemicals that damage the vessel wall and factors that cause clotting and destruction of muscle and collagen in the vessel wall. This whole process is called vascular — or endothelial — inflammation.

It is not like inflammation of a joint with pain and swelling and redness. Yet, it resembles inflammation in other ways. Destructive cells and chemicals invade the endothelium and disrupt the architecture.

Today we have medications that can stop and even reverse this inflammatory process. These medications are called statins and other anti-cholesterol medicines called fibrates, the medicines that fight insulin resistance (TZDs — Thia-zolidine-diones) and the blood pressure reducers — Angiotensin Converting Enzyme (ACE) Inhibitors, Angiotensin Receptor Blockers (ARBs), Beta Blockers, Calcium Channel Blockers and Alpha Blockers.

6

TESTS FOR THE
METABOLIC SYNDROME

If you suspect you have the metabolic syndrome, or think you may be at risk for developing it, you need the following tests. Ask your doctor to order them for you, then make an appointment to review the results.

Even if you have diabetes, you may not have *any* symptoms. You may blame vague symptoms, such as tiredness, on stress or overwork.

1. **Blood chemistry** panel measures blood urea nitrogen (BUN) and creatinine to evaluate kidney function; sodium, potassium, chloride to evaluate hydration, kidney disease, drug effects, and other important conditions; serum proteins to evaluate nutrition, liver function, immunity; liver enzymes to evaluate liver health and drug effects; blood uric acid to detect gout and vascular inflammation.
2. **Urinalysis** to detect kidney disease and infection. It will also detect micro-albumin, a very important predictor of heart and kidney disease in the metabolic syndrome and in diabetes.
3. **Cholesterol analysis** to include total cholesterol, triglycerides, LDL-C and HDL-C.

4. **Advanced cholesterol analysis** can be of great value to decide which drugs are indicated for cholesterol management. It can also reveal whether other types of lipid abnormalities are present such as VLDL (very low density lipoproteins). Additionally, it can show how much of the "good" cholesterol (HDL) is really good and how much of the "bad" cholesterol (LDL) is really bad.

5. **A blood cell count** to rule out abnormalities in red cells, white cells and platelets which might reveal anemia, leukemia, infection, bleeding tendencies or other unsuspected problems.

6. **A chest X-ray** to check the size of the heart, condition of lungs and bone structure and to find unexpected abnormalities, like tuberculosis.

7. **An electrocardiogram (EKG)** to check heart size, rhythm, disease.

8. **An echocardiogram (ultrasound)** to check heart size, condition of heart valves, and the heart's pumping ability.

9. **A treadmill** or other heart stress test if #1 and #2 are abnormal, followed by an angiogram, if the stress test is not normal.

10. **Ultrasound** of the carotid arteries, the kidney arteries and the arteries in the legs. Partial blockage may exist already and may influence decisions about which drugs to use for blood pressure control and cholesterol management.

11. **Inflammatory markers** such as C-Reactive Protein, tumor necrosis factor, and others can be measured to indicate the extent of the inflammation and how to treat it. Diabetes and the metabolic syndrome are both conditions in which the blood vessels are being damaged by inflammation.

12. **Fasting blood glucose** levels and the glucose levels measured one, two and three hours after drinking 75 grams of

glucose, will usually distinguish normal individuals from those with metabolic syndrome and those who have diabetes *(Fig. 3)*.

"Do-It-Yourself" Preliminary Testing

Are you afraid of going to the doctor? Are the lab tests too expensive?

If so, there are some things you can do for yourself. Try this:

Have a diabetic friend or family member test your blood sugar with their home testing monitor. Remember, to get an accurate reading, you must take the blood test **two hours after eating.** If your blood sugar is above 140 mg/dl, you are glucose intolerant. If your blood sugar is over 180 mg/dl, you are already diabetic.

For even more proof, go to your pharmacy and purchase a hemoglobin A1c test kit — about $25. This shows what your blood sugar has been for the past 90 days. It is a simple finger stick test that measures how much red pigment in the red blood cells (hemoglobin) has combined with glucose — the normal level is 4–6%.

If your results are greater than 6%, you have either metabolic syndrome or diabetes. Over 8%, you are already diabetic. Make an appointment with your doctor immediately.

PLEASE NOTE: This "do-it-yourself" test is not meant as a substitute for good medical care.

7

BEYOND DIET AND EXERCISE:

Understanding the Medications

Treatment should begin with a thorough medical examination to determine your ability to exercise safely and to measure each part of the metabolic syndrome:

1. High blood pressure
2. Cholesterol abnormalities
3. Insulin resistance
4. Obesity — especially waist measurement

> **EAT WISELY, EXERCISE AND TAKE NECESSARY MEDICATIONS — *WAITING* IS *NOT* AN OPTION IN PREVENTING TYPE 2 DIABETES**

Lifestyle changes are absolutely necessary. The changes must be permanent, lifelong, and uninterrupted.

The fact is that few succeed at maintaining lifestyle changes even though many try. Lack of commitment, peer pressure, cultural and racial customs, and anxiety and depression all get in the way of making permanent and necessary lifestyle changes.

Easy to start — hard to maintain. The initial enthusiasm for a diet wears off. There is always a ready excuse to indulge — birthdays, weddings, holidays, and even funerals.

We live in an "eat-eat-eat" culture. We reward ourselves and our children with food. We try to relieve stress with food. We eat when we are happy, angry, tired or bored.

> The raging debate about which diet is best for losing weight and reversing the cholesterol problem can be cut short: Eat less and exercise more. Combine push-ups with push-aways...from the table.

Generally, it is smarter to start exercise gradually and work up to more strenuous exertion. You can't go from sitting on the couch to climbing Mt. Kilimanjaro in one day!

Start with walking or a combination of walking and short periods of jogging. Mow the lawn, rake leaves, weed the garden, trim the shrubbery, vacuum the house. Move around faster. Ride a bike. Walk the dog. Park farther from the store. Take the stairs.

If you are out of shape, buy an exercise video. Start with low-impact exercises. Jump rope. Swim. Dance. Try push-ups. Join a yoga class. Join a gym, or hire a personal trainer. Get moving — every day!

A Patient Tells About "The Weight Escape"

When my husband passed away, I was left to raise four young children by myself. Fortunately, he had left us enough money so I didn't have to work outside the home. But I was grieving and depressed, and the anxiety of starting my life over frightened me — especially the thought of dating.

So, I ate and ate.

I know now that subconsciously I ate to make myself so fat and unattractive no one would want to date me. Gaining weight was an escape for me.

I succeeded in insulating myself from life and stayed busy raising my children.

Eventually I went to the doctor because my back hurt. He told me it was from the weight. As it turned out, my weight had caused more than back problems. I had high blood pressure, and the doctor wanted to test me for type 2 diabetes. My father had died from complications of diabetes at the age of 54. That scared me, even though I felt fine.

Tests showed that my cholesterol was high, but my blood sugar wasn't high enough to be diabetic. The doctor said I had the metabolic syndrome with insulin-resistance, and if I would take medications for blood pressure and cholesterol and something to make me produce better insulin, I probably wouldn't become diabetic. And I had to lose weight and exercise.

"Watch those carbohydrates," he told me. He said metabolic syndrome is serious. It was hard for me to believe that I could have a heart attack or stroke if I continued my current lifestyle.

I took the medications religiously. I must admit, I often failed at the diet and exercise. In spite of that, a surprising thing happened. When I went to see my doctor — even though I had only lost a few pounds — my blood pressure was normal, and the blood tests came back showing a big improvement in my cholesterol.

I hate to admit this. I felt like I cheated, but succeeded at the same time. I promised to diet and exercise, but it's so hard. Even though I know I sometimes eat too many carbs, I never forget my medications. I really am trying to live a healthier life. And I do want to live to see my children grown — and grandkids, too!

Margaret S., Phoenix, AZ

START MEDICATIONS EARLY — ALONG WITH LIFESTYLE CHANGES

There are hundreds of books, pamphlets and promotions claiming to know all the answers, often giving conflicting advice. Beware of those that encourage you *NOT* to take the proven prescriptions, but instead suggest supplements and herbal remedies — especially the ones *they* sell.

ARE THE MEDICATIONS SAFE?

"But," you may say, "I don't like taking pills. I only want *natural* products."

The statins, fibrates and nicotinic acid used to correct cholesterol abnormalities, the ACE inhibitors and ARBs and other medications for blood pressure control have a very good safety record. Similarly, the TZDs, used to reduce insulin resistance, are safe when prescribed appropriately. These medications are discussed in detail in the following chapter.

Exceptions: An allergic reaction to any medication is unpredictable. But the majority of reactions are minor; they usually occur early on and stop when the medication is no longer taken.

The statins may rarely cause muscle injury (rhabdomyolysis). The problem is easily solved when the patient reports aches and pains to the physician, and the medication is stopped.

Liver injury is rare. It is easily detected, however, by blood tests. Injury is reversed by stopping the medication. Your doctor will assess the blood tests and decide what is best for you.

Large doses and certain combinations of medications may cause problems but, again, if you report side effects early to your doctor, and medication is stopped or changed, then no permanent harm results.

Prescribed drugs may clash with some herbal remedies and supplements, with other medications, and even certain foods — like grapefruit juice. Such incompatibilities may determine how well a prescribed medication works, how its action may be blocked or how side effects are increased, so it is necessary to tell your doctor about *all* prescriptions, supplements and over-the-counter medications you are taking. Your doctor can then decide which medications to prescribe for you.

IMPORTANT POINTS

• Package inserts for prescription medicines are required by law to list all *possible* side effects and may present an unbalanced view.

Remember: The medications recommended for the metabolic syndrome and for diabetes have a great track record. Their benefits outweigh the risks many times over!

• If your blood pressure is usually 160/90 mmHg, exercise may raise it temporarily to 190/100. It may not return to 160/90 quickly. During that period of really high blood pressure, your risk of a stroke or heart attack is higher, especially if you already have damaged arteries. High pressure can also cause retinal hemorrhage or retinal separation. *This is why you must have a thorough medical exam before starting an exercise program.*

• In the long run, exercise and weight loss will lower your blood pressure, but not always to the desired normal 130/80 mmHg. It is wise to get a thorough medical evaluation and to start blood pressure medication early (if indicated) before starting a vigorous exercise program.

• It is important to note that some kinds of high blood pressure will *never* come down with exercise and weight loss. An example is the high blood pressure caused by a narrow kidney artery (renal stenosis). That is why you should have a kidney ultrasound test before you start making lifestyle changes.

• If you do have renal artery stenosis, some medications like ACE inhibitors, which are used to treat high blood pressure, may harm you. The kidney artery should be ballooned open first and may have to be kept open by a stent. If so, your doctor may decide to increase the medication dosage. Always consult your medical advisor before changing medications and dosage or adding/omitting supplements.

• While you wait for exercise and weight loss to improve your health, the untreated high blood pressure and cholesterol abnormalities continue to damage arteries. This is especially true if you do not remain committed to lifestyle changes. Medications will protect you while you diet and exercise to lose weight.

• Treatment should begin with the thorough medical examination described earlier. Each part of the metabolic syndrome should be considered separately and treated effectively:
  – High blood pressure
  – Cholesterol abnormalities
  – Insulin resistance
  – Obesity

The medical examination will determine if it is safe for you to start vigorous exercises, like jogging or running. Remember, your heart's coronary arteries may be partially clogged already. That is why the EKG, the echocardiogram and the heart stress test are extremely important.

EXERCISE AND WEIGHT LOSS
  • Improve cholesterol abnormalities
  • Reduce blood pressure
  • Decrease insulin resistance

But, it may take a long time to reach your goals. This is part of the reason why it is important to combine medications with your diet and exercise plan. **Medications not only help you reach your goals faster; they can also protect you against a disastrous heart attack or stroke.**

**IT IS WISE TO IMPLEMENT
LIFESTYLE CHANGES AND MEDICATIONS
AT THE SAME TIME.
WAITING IS NOT AN OPTION.**

A Family Affair

I met her in the hospital after her heart attack at age 42. An elevated blood sugar was found with readings above 300 mg/dl on several occasions.

During my consultation, I explained to her that she was diabetic.

"You know, it's funny; my mother told me I would never become a diabetic because no one in our family had it," she said.

After discussing her family history, I commented on the fact that her uncle had died in his fifties and had perhaps been diabetic.

She countered, saying her grandmother had told her he only had "bad sugar."

"He died of a heart attack — not diabetes," she said. Continuing, she added, "I was told 15 years ago while I was pregnant with my second child that I had diabetes. But the doctor said it was 'gestational diabetes' and would go away after I delivered the baby. It did, and I didn't worry any more."

I asked about the birth weight of the baby, and she laughed.

"Nine pounds. A really healthy baby!"

She admitted that after pregnancy she continued to gain weight, reaching 180 pounds when she weighed herself at her doctor's office two weeks before this current hospitalization.

"Why were you visiting the doctor?" I asked.

"I was concerned about my weight and had read how unhealthy it was. The nurse told me I was okay — just overweight. She said my blood pressure was 'a little up' — 145/80 — but not enough to take medication."

"Did they do blood tests?" I asked.

"Only the blood sugar," she said. "And they told me it was okay. I think it was, like 110, and I remember the nurse saying it was way before the level for diabetes, so I didn't need to worry."

"Do you remember if that was fasting blood sugar?" I asked.

"Yes," she replied. "I hadn't had anything to eat or drink for 12 hours."

Her son was sitting in the corner of her hospital room. I judged he was about 15 and probably the one who had weighed nine pounds at birth. He was obviously overweight.

"Have you had your son checked for diabetes?" I asked.

"Yes, last year when he went out for sports, he had a physical. They took blood and said he was okay."

"Was he heavy then, also?" I asked.

"Oh, yes," she said. "He was going out for football and the coach wanted him to be big."

"What about your first child?" I asked.

"He's fine," she said. "He's 18 now and a track star — he's a runner. He's always outside doing something. He's really active. But this one," motioning to her son, "he plays computer games all day. He hates being outdoors. Except for football. He loves playing football. And he's big. The rest of the time, he's in front of the TV or the computer."

Then I asked her about brothers and sisters.

"I have one sister — no brothers. My sister is heavy, too. She's three years younger than me. She's married, but can't have children. She said her doctor told her something about cysts on her ovaries. The doctor told my sister she might have some hormone problems. She has hair on her chin, and she's only had a few periods in her whole life."

"Has she ever been treated for diabetes?" I asked.

"Yes, she has. I think it was about 2 months ago when the doctor told her she was borderline on sugar and needed to lose weight. She and I were planning to go on a diet together, but I ended up here with this heart attack."

I saw her daily after that first examination, because she had to undergo triple coronary bypass surgery, and her blood sugars had to be controlled very closely. She left the hospital about a week after the bypass surgery and scheduled an appointment to see me in the office a week later.

Her husband came with her to my office. When we sat down to talk he said, "Tell the doctor about your mother's cooking and how she brought you treats when you got home."

It was hard to believe what she told me. She said her mother believed that "when you have diabetes, you can't use sugar properly, so you have to eat more of it to get it into your cells." She continued, "Mom brought my favorite 3-layer chocolate cake with fudgy frosting and a plateful of my favorite chocolate chip cookies and a jar of honey. She told me that honey was okay to use, because it's a natural *sweetener."*

This story is typical of many diabetics and their families. During the rest of her office visit, I explained some of her misconceptions:

1.   *The patient's diabetes was diagnosed at the time of her heart attack. Actually, she had diabetes during her second pregnancy and should have been warned to lose weight and to have tests at least every six months for metabolic syndrome (weight, waist, cholesterol, blood pressure). Then she should have been placed on cardio-protective medications and urged to make heart-protective lifestyle changes.*

2.   *Gestational diabetes occurs in about one of four pregnancies and is more prevalent in Hispanic and African American women. It usually disappears after the baby is delivered, but the mother will always have a predisposition toward diabetes and will need to watch her weight and keep active. She will need to be vigilant and be carefully monitored for type 2 diabetes.*

3.   *Her 9-pound baby is typical of diabetic mothers. That baby grew up obese at 15, with all the external marks of metabolic syndrome. He is heading for diabetes, and at his young age, already has fatty deposits in his arteries. Being encouraged to gain even more weight for sports is very wrong. He should be placed on a strict weight loss and exercise program, possibly with cholesterol-lowering medications.*

4.   *Relatives, like her uncle, who die early, should be suspected of having diabetes. Even if no proof can be found, the entire family should be observed for metabolic syndrome and diabetes.*

5.   *This patient's visit to her doctor a few weeks before her heart attack illustrates two common mistakes. First, her blood pressure was definitely elevated and her fasting blood sugar was definitely in the "insulin resistant" range. Second, in addition to a referral to a dietician for weight loss, she should have been*

placed on blood pressure medication immediately, *and she should have had a cholesterol evaluation, an EKG and the other tests described in the text for evaluating metabolic syndrome.*

6. *Her sister has "polycystic ovary syndrome," a condition in which the ovaries are filled with cysts, the person is obese, and has all the marks of metabolic syndrome and type 2 diabetes. She needs much more than dietary counseling.*
   *The word **"borderline"** should never be used in describing a blood sugar level. If there is uncertainty, retesting of fasting and after-meal sugars or even a glucose tolerance test is appropriate and* urgent. *Diabetes is like pregnancy: it is **never** borderline.*

7. *After discharge from the hospital, this woman received terribly wrong advice from her mother and incorrect information about honey. Diabetics are unable to process sugar, but they certainly do not need more of it! Sugar is sugar. Honey is a sugar and should be used sparingly. This patient suffered from a sad lack of family support and misinformation about diabetes.*

8. *The good news is that the hospitalization and heart attack scared this patient into revising her diet and exercise plan. She did lose weight, has started on appropriate medication, and has had a positive influence on her overweight son and sister.*

8

TREATING CHOLESTEROL ABNORMALITIES

The metabolic syndrome is identified by these triglyceride and cholesterol abnormalities:

- triglycerides higher than 150 mg/dl
- HDL-C below 50 mg/dl
- LDL-C consisting of small particles

A combination low fat diet and exercise program can significantly correct cholesterol abnormalities. However, only a small portion of cholesterol in our bodies comes from food. Most cholesterol is manufactured by the liver, so medications are essential and should be started early in the prevention program, in addition to dietary changes and an exercise program.

■ Medications for Treating Triglyceride and Cholesterol Abnormalities

The medications that improve cholesterol abnormalities include the **Statins**, the **Fibrates, Niacin, Bile Acid Sequestrants** and **Omega-3 Fatty Acids.**

STATIN drugs lower total cholesterol, raise HDL-C, decrease triglycerides and lower LDL-C.

The statins inhibit an enzyme necessary for the formation of cholesterol in the liver. When the liver is less preoccupied with making cholesterol, it can clear LDL-C (bad cholesterol) from the circulation more efficiently. It is thought that LDL-C reduction contributes significantly toward keeping blood vessels healthy and results in fewer cardiovascular events such as heart attacks and strokes.

It is also believed that the statins are beneficial because they reduce vascular inflammation. When statins act on endothelial cells, they increase nitric oxide (NO) formation, which is very necessary for the normal structure and function of blood vessels. Nitric oxide prevents blood vessels from becoming narrow structurally and from closing down in response to sympathetic nerve stimulation, as in periods of stress. Statins also reduce the tendency of blood to clot.

These benefits of statins go beyond lowering the cholesterol levels. When patients resist taking statins, telling their doctor that they would rather try weight loss and exercise to reduce cholesterol, they are either forgetting or perhaps do not understand that statins do much more than lower cholesterol.

> *Statins actually restore the health of blood vessels.*

There is evidence that statins stabilize vulnerable plaques by stimulating the formation of a thick cap over the plaque. This prevents plaque rupture and the catastrophic consequences of plaque rupture such as heart attacks and strokes *(See Fig. 4 and Fig. 6)*. This is one of the most important reasons to use statins early in the metabolic syndrome.

The statins currently in use are Lipitor (atorvastatin), Zocor (simvistatin), Pravachol (pravastatin), Mevacor (lovastatin), Lescol (fluvastatin) and Crestor (rosuvistatin). The choice of a statin is often dictated by price as well as prescription benefit plans. All statins have LDL-C and triglyceride-lowering powers and all raise HDL-C modestly.

Pravachol and Lescol offer another special advantage. They are processed in the liver by pathways not used by other drugs. Therefore, they are less likely to raise or lower the blood levels of other drugs such as the antibiotics Erythromycin, Biaxin and Zithromax commonly used for infections. These antibiotics (Erythromycin, Biaxin and Zithromax) are known to increase to toxic levels if used in combination with Lipitor, Zocor and Mevacor, even to the point of causing sudden death. Check with your doctor about mixing cholesterol-lowering drugs with other medications.

> **RX WARNING:**
> If you are taking Lipitor, Zocor and Mevacor
> **AVOID**
> Zithromax, Biaxin and Erythromycin.
> **CONSULT WITH YOUR DOCTOR.**

The side effects of statins are generally mild and may include nausea, fatigue, rashes, diarrhea, flatulence and myalgia or aching muscles. Most side effects are often temporary and may disappear with continued use.

One rare, but occasionally life-threatening, side effect is rhabdomyolysis, which means "muscle breakdown." The affected individual experiences severe, generalized muscle pains, often with fever. Fortunately, if the statin is stopped immediately, no permanent harm results and recovery is rapid. The public has been somewhat over-sensitized to this reaction by publicity and package-insert warnings. Consequently, doctors often experience patients' resistance when they attempt to prescribe statins.

Also, at the first sign of a muscle ache or pain, even if localized and unrelated to the medication, some patients will stop the statin and reject any suggestion that they try a different statin.

This is a bad decision because statins are very important protectors of blood vessels. Every major study, from Scandinavia to Great Britain and the United States, has shown great reductions in the incidence of heart attacks and strokes when statins are used.

An oddity most patients seem to know about is that grapefruit juice can increase the risk of muscle problems. This is because the grapefruit juice and statins follow the same path through the liver. Grapefruit juice blocks the liver's ability to process the statins, making the concentration of statins rise and thereby causing muscle pains.

It is important that patients ask their physicians to check all their medications before prescribing statins to avoid medication clashes. Many physicians ask each new patient to bag up and bring into the office every prescription medication, herbal supplement and over-the-counter formulation that they take. This "brown bag check-up" is much more accurate than a list of medications, and it allows the physician to check for incompatibilities and improper dosing and directions.

Statins should be avoided during pregnancy and in patients with pre-existing liver disease. They have not been used in children but, with the increasing incidence of childhood obesity and pre-diabetes, the use of statins in this age group is under re-evaluation.

When patients are started on statins, it is recommended that liver enzymes be measured about every two months for six months and less often thereafter. Although this rarely happens, if the enzyme levels rise to three times normal, the statin must be stopped.

Patient behavior here is opposite that seen with muscle pains. They "forget" to come in for liver enzyme checks, particularly if there are no symptoms. Therefore, physicians should not prescribe statins for more than 30 days initially, so that patients will not receive automatic renewals without being monitored.

Regrettably, many prescription plans require doctors to write 90-day prescriptions, which runs contrary to the best interests of patients who are receiving statins initially on a trial basis.

> **Statins can be used in combination with other cholesterol-lowering medications, but careful monitoring is necessary because certain combinations may increase muscle and liver problems.**

FIBRATES (FIBRIC ACID DERIVATIVES)

FIBRATES are very helpful medications because they slow the production of fatty acids by fat cells throughout the body and especially those in the abdomen. When the liver is not required to process these fatty acids, it can make more of the good cholestrol, the HDL.

Fibrates are potent reducers of triglycerides, and they raise HDL-C more than statins do. When fibrates and statins are used in combination, the HDL-C (an important protector of blood vessels) can be raised significantly.

The fibrates are marketed under various brands. One of them is Tricor (fenofibrate), which also lowers the LDL-C. Some of the other fibrates include Lopid (gemfibrozol) and Atromid-S (clofibrate), and the newest one, Antara (fenofibrate).

Liver enzymes and renal function should be carefully monitored. Side effects are generally mild and temporary, but fibrates can cause gallstones. These medications should always be used under medical supervision.

Fibrates are especially useful for lowering triglycerides and are therefore good agents to use in the metabolic syndrome and diabetes, particularly since they also raise HDL-C. This is important

Endothelial Inflammation: How Statins Work

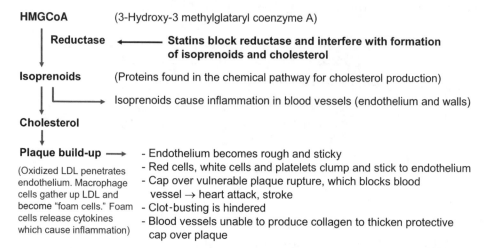

HMGCoA   (3-Hydroxy-3 methylglataryl coenzyme A)

| Reductase ◄——— **Statins block reductase and interfere with formation of isoprenoids and cholesterol**

Isoprenoids   (Proteins found in the chemical pathway for cholesterol production)

| └———► Isoprenoids cause inflammation in blood vessels (endothelium and walls)

Cholesterol
↓

Plaque build-up ——►   - Endothelium becomes rough and sticky
(Oxidized LDL penetrates   - Red cells, white cells and platelets clump and stick to endothelium
endothelium. Macrophage   - Cap over vulnerable plaque rupture, which blocks blood
cells gather up LDL and   vessel → heart attack, stroke
become "foam cells." Foam - Clot-busting is hindered
cells release cytokines   - Blood vessels unable to produce collagen to thicken protective
which cause inflammation)   cap over plaque

Statins (Lipitor, Crestor, Pravachol, Lescol, Zocor) are HMGCoA reductase inhibitors. This inhibition blocks both cholesterol production and inflammation. The anti-inflammatory effects of statins are important reasons to take statins and to continue them even when ideal cholesterol numbers have been reached.

Figure 5

because most people with the metabolic syndrome have low HDL-C levels, and the HDL-C carries away LDL-C and other cholesterol particles to the liver.

Tricor and Antara (fenofibrates) reduce LDL-C and, importantly, are thought to change small LDL-C particles into larger ones which are less harmful to blood vessels. Tricor and Antara also reduce Lp(a), a protein responsible for arterial disease.

When fibrates are used in conjunction with statins, side effects may increase, particularly muscle problems. Fibrates are not recommended for pregnant women, children, or patients with pre-existing liver and kidney disease.

> *Lifestyle changes do not increase HDL-C*
> *(the "good" cholesterol) significantly.*
> *It is therefore very important that*
> *appropriate medications be started early*
> *and not be avoided. They should be*
> *continued without interruption and should*
> *be closely monitored by your doctor.*

NIACIN (NICOTINIC ACID)

Niacin, one of the B vitamins, raises HDL-C and lowers triglycerides, LDL-C and Lp(a). It can interfere with blood sugar control, but it may be used for diabetics if adjustments are made.

Some formulations, however, may prolong the presence of niacin in the circulation to such an extent that daily doses lead to accumulation and liver toxicity. A patient needs to remain under a doctor's supervision and have periodic blood tests in order to assess liver function.

Niacin's chief drawback is that some patients experience flushing and itching. Others tolerate niacin well. Patients should be aware that most over-the-counter niacin preparations, such as the fast-acting formulations which cost less than the prescription drug, are generally ineffective. They should also be aware that the so-called "non-flushing formulations" contain nicotinamide, not niacin, and are therefore not effective.

The preferred formulation is Niaspan in doses up to 2 grams daily. When the nicotinic acid is given in a slow-release form such as Niaspan, flushing is less common. Flushing can be minimized by taking the Niaspan with a meal, by avoiding spicy foods and alcohol at that meal and by taking an uncoated aspirin 30 minutes to an hour before the Niaspan. Since many patients are already taking the "baby aspirin" (81 mg) for cardiovascular health, they should be allowed to change to an uncoated form of aspirin, to be taken 30 minutes to an hour before the Niaspan and the meal.

Another formulation, Advicor, is a combination of niacin and Lovostatin.

ZETIA (EZETIMIBE)

Zetia is a cholesterol-lowering agent which blocks cholesterol absorption from the intestine. Alone or with a statin, Zetia will reduce total cholesterol, LDL-C and triglycerides while it raises the HDL-C.

The incidence of side effects is low, although intestinal discomfort, nausea and backache have been reported. The chief reasons to use Zetia are to achieve goals for cholesterol and triglyceride reduction without increasing statin doses to such a high level that they might cause muscle problems, and also to avoid statin and fibrate combinations which may further increase side effects.

Zetia (ezetimibe) can be taken as a 10 mg tablet in combination with any statin, or it can be taken as Vytorin which is a combination of Zocor and Zetia (simvistatin and ezetimibe).

BILE ACID SEQUESTRANTS

These medications act within the intestine where they bind bile acids and interfere with their absorption. Bile acid concentration within the liver cells is subsequently reduced; cholesterol is converted more rapidly into bile acid; and the concentration of cholesterol in liver cells falls. The liver cells will then accept more LDL-C, clearing even more LDL-C from the circulation. Some reduction also occurs in VLDL-C.

Unfortunately, however, triglyceride levels also become elevated, limiting the use of bile acid sequestrants in the metabolic syndrome and diabetes. They may cause a lot of intestinal discomfort and interfere with the absorption of some vitamins and medications.

Drugs in this class are Questran, Colestid, and Welchol. They may decrease the absorption of important medications like Lasix (furosemide), thiazides, tetracycline and penicillin. They may also disturb important heart medications like digitalis and verapamil. Your physician should be aware of these potential clashes.

OMEGA-3 FATTY ACIDS

Omega-3 fatty acids, found in fish, flaxseed, canola oil and walnuts, cannot be manufactured by the body and therefore must be obtained from food or supplements. These fatty acids lower the triglycerides, lower blood pressure, reduce inflammation in blood vessels, prevent fatal heart rhythm disturbances and act as anti-clotting agents.

They should be included in the diet or added as a capsule supplement because they protect the heart and blood vessels. They have been shown to raise LDL-C modestly, which is a potentially harmful result, but LDL-C is not elevated in patients with the metabolic syndrome and the increase may not be significant.

Two 6-oz. servings of fish per week is the general recommendation for most adults. Good sources of the Omega-3 fatty acids include:

- salmon
- herring
- tuna
- sardines
- haddock
- mackerel
- shrimp
- crabmeat
- flounder
- halibut
- catfish
- pollock

Certain fish should be avoided because of high mercury content. These include shark, swordfish, and albacore. However, salmon, shrimp, pollock, canned light tuna, and catfish are relatively low in mercury content.

Omega-3 fatty acids are available without prescription from pharmacies and health food stores. Three 1-gram capsules should be taken daily, either in a single dose, or as 1-gram three times a day. These capsules should be taken with food. If they are refrigerated, there is less chance of "burping." Some brands advertise "no burping" and "no fishy smell."

Omega-3 fatty acids are available in a highly purified form in Omacor, which does require a prescription. Four 1-gram capsules daily is the recommended dosage.

It should be noted that Omega-3 fatty acids in capsule form do not interfere with other medications. They can be taken with statins and other cholesterol-lowering medications, and with any diabetic and blood pressure medications.

A Riches-to-Rags Story

The couple was wealthy and well-travelled. They decided to retire in the warmth of Arizona where they lived in opulent surroundings and enjoyed a country club lifestyle. She was a wonderful hostess. She had taken classes at Le Cordon Bleu in Paris and prepared gourmet meals.

Her cream-laden foods and dazzling desserts, however, were completely unsuited to his condition.

He was a diabetic. He was overweight, suffered from high blood sugar, high blood pressure and high cholesterol. But he had no will power and would not change his eating habits nor take the necessary medications regularly. He did not manage his blood sugar well, either.

I pleaded with him to control his diabetes and take medication to prevent cardiovascular disasters, but to no avail.

As time passed, his wife died, leaving him to care for himself. Continuing the same irresponsible attitude he had always shown toward his diabetes, he ultimately suffered a stroke which left him paralyzed on the right side and with a significant speech problem.

This required prolonged nursing home care and rehabilitation, becoming very costly. After several years of nursing home care, he had spent all of his fortune and ended up living in the home of someone who had taken pity on him.

He was penniless and died a pauper.

This story exemplifies the enormous physical suffering and financial devastation that diabetes can cause.

9

TREATING ELEVATED BLOOD PRESSURE IN THE METABOLIC SYNDROME

Before beginning treatment for elevated blood pressure, for your own safety and to establish baseline measurements, ask your doctor to order:

- A kidney ultrasound to rule out kidney artery narrowing (renal stenosis)
- Blood tests to assess kidney function (specifically levels of the waste products, blood urea nitrogen — BUN — and creatinine)
- A urinalysis to measure protein and micro-albumin levels

> **The Goal: Blood pressure should be 130/80 mmHg.**

No one "owns" a fixed set of numbers. Blood pressure fluctuates with stress, relaxation, sleep, exercise — with ordinary daily living. Some readings will be higher than 130/80 and some will be lower. What is really important is that most readings taken at different times of the day — and under different circumstances — should be between 100 to 130 systolic and 60 and 80 diastolic.

Now that you understand the possible fluctuations, you can see how the occasional reading done in the doctor's office gives an incomplete picture.

If you can buy a blood pressure monitor (about $40 at most drug stores), you will get a much better assessment of your blood pressure. Keep a record of your pressure, and take the record with you to your periodic appointments so your doctor can assess the readings.

Be advised that the "blood pressure monitors" set out for public use in many stores and pharmacies may be inaccurate since children often play with the equipment. Results are much more accurate with your own monitor. Ask your doctor or pharmacist to show you how to use it properly.

BLOOD PRESSURE MEDICATIONS

There are several classes of blood pressure medications. The five medications listed below are used most often, usually two or three in combination with one another. Understanding what these medications are and how some of them work in partnership can help patients and their families ensure that the medications are taken properly and regularly.

- Angiotensin Converting Enzyme (ACE) Inhibitors
- Angiotensin Receptor Blockers (ARBs)
- Beta Blockers
- Calcium Channel Blockers
- Diuretics
- Aldosterone Antagonists

ACE INHIBITORS AND ARBs

In both the metabolic syndrome and in diabetes, the ACE inhibitors and ARBs are preferred medications because they lower blood pressure as well as protect the kidneys.

The generic names of the ACE inhibitors all end with the letters "PRIL," like lisinopril, ramipril, captopril, benazapril and many others.

The generic names of ARBs end in the letters "SARTAN," like olmesartan, candesartan, valsartan, losartan, irbesartan and many others.

Sometimes ACE inhibitors and ARBs are combined with a diuretic, usually Hydrochlorothiazide (HCTZ). Some combinations include Hyzaar, Benicar-HCT, Diovan-HCT, and Avalide. These combinations can improve blood pressure control.

ACE inhibitors block the formation of a chemical called Angiotensin II, a nasty agent that narrows blood vessels, increases blood clotting, causes endothelial inflammation, contributes to stickiness of cells (especially platelets) and often interferes with the entry of glucose into cells.

Recent work has shown that Angiotensin II is especially bad when it attaches to receptors on blood vessels *(see Fig. 5)*. It causes increased clotting, blood vessel narrowing and elevated blood pressure. The ARBs block the attachment of Angiotensin II to receptors, hence their name, Angiotensin Receptor Blockers.

Therefore, ACE inhibitors and ARBs, by acting against Angiotensin II and its attachment to receptors, not only lower blood pressure, but they also reduce clotting, inflammation and vasoconstriction or narrowing of blood vessels. They also help glucose to enter cells.

> ACE inhibitors and ARBs are so important in delaying the progress of kidney disease that they should probably be used in all patients with albumin in the urine, even if these patients are not yet hypertensive.

ACE inhibitors and ARBs have shown themselves capable of preventing kidney damage and even reversing any existing damage. They have also become important for heart protection, especially when a patient is in heart failure or has suffered a heart attack.

The Origin and Actions of Angiotensin II and the Locations Where Drugs Act

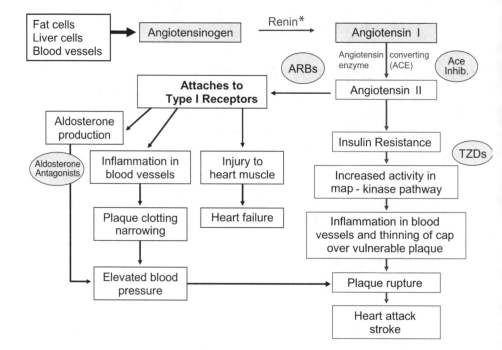

The Renin-Angiotensin-Aldosterone System (RAAS)

ACE Inhibitors - Block conversion of Angiotensin I to Angiotensin II

ARBs - (Angiotensin receptor blockers) Hinder attachment of Angiotensin II to receptors

TZDs - (Thia-zolidine-diones) Decrease insulin resistance

Aldosterone Antagonists - Diminish aldosterone production

* Renin Inhibitors - New drugs currently undergoing FDA approval

Figure 6

DRAWBACKS TO USING ACE INHIBITORS AND ARBs

ACE inhibitors can sometimes cause a troublesome, dry, irritating cough, caused by an accumulation of bradykinin in the lungs. Bradykinin is a chemical that is beneficial to blood vessels by keeping the endothelium healthy. This cough goes away when the medications are stopped. If the cough is very troublesome, consult with your doctor, but do not stop medications on your own.

Rarely, ACE inhibitors and ARBs may cause swelling of the lips and tongue (angio-edema). They are not recommended for use during pregnancy.

They should not be used with arthritis medications if kidney function is abnormal. These arthritis medications include popular, over-the-counter drugs like Advil, Aleve, Ibuprofen, as well as prescribed medications like Naprosyn and Celebrex. Consult with your doctor before taking these medications.

BETA BLOCKERS

Beta blockers *block* those nerves in the heart and blood vessels responsible for increasing the heart rate and for narrowing blood vessels. When the beta nerves are blocked, blood vessels relax and the heart rate slows down. Beta blockers have *nothing* to do with the insulin-producing beta cells in the pancreas.

The generic names of the beta blockers all end in "OL," like metoprolol, carvedilol, atenolol, bisoprolol, propranalol and many others.

Beta blockers are often prescribed with diuretics and with ACE inhibitors and ARBs. Beta blockers are especially useful after heart attacks when they have been shown to prevent heart failure, rhythm disturbances of the heart, and further heart attacks.

Carvedilol is especially useful in the metabolic syndrome because it preserves insulin sensitivity, does not lower HDL-C, and does not increase LDL-C. Most other beta blockers increase insulin resistance and affect HDL-C and LDL-C unfavorably.

Some beta blockers have been reported to make breathing more difficult for patients with asthma and emphysema. More recently, this idea has been challenged, and certain beta blockers, like carvedilol, seem to be well tolerated by patients with breathing problems. You and your doctor can discuss these possibilities.

CALCIUM CHANNEL BLOCKERS (CCBs)

The Calcium Channel Blockers (CCBs) lower blood pressure by blocking the flow of calcium into the muscle of blood vessels, thereby causing the blood vessels to relax and dilate. This reduces the resistance to the flow of blood and eases the work of the heart muscle. By blocking the entry of calcium into the heart muscle itself, CCBs are useful in treating rhythm problems of the heart. On the other hand, CCBs may block electrical flow from the top of the heart to the bottom and slow the heart too much.

CCBs are divided into two classes:
1. The Nondihydropyridines which act on the heart muscle as well as blood vessels.
   They are Diltiazem SR (Slow Release), also known as Cardizem SR. Diltiazem CD is also known as Cardizem CD or Dilacor XR or Tiazac.
   Verapamil LA (Long Acting) is also called Calan SR, Covera HS, Isoptin SR and Verelan.
2. The Dihydropyridines:
   These are Norvasc (amlodipine), DynaCirc CR (Controlled Release) (isradipine), Sular (nisoldipine), Cardene SR (nicardipine).
   The generic names of the Dihydropines all end in "PINE."
   They may be preferred for the treatment of high blood pressure because they act primarily on blood vessels rather than the heart muscle.
   In pre-diabetes and diabetes, they improve the flow of blood through the kidneys.

In pre-diabetes and diabetes, ACE inhibitors, ARBs and certain beta blockers, such as Coreg (carvedilol) are preferred as initial therapy.

If target blood pressure is not reached with these agents, CCBs of the Dihydropyridine class can be added for further blood pressure reduction while preserving heart muscle function and electrical conduction.

Norvasc (amlodipine) may cause ankle swelling. This can be reversed by adding an ACE inhibitor (benazepril) to amlodipine in a tablet called Lotrel.

The calcium channel blockers can be used with ACE inhibitors, ARBs and beta blockers. Like beta blockers, they can change the electrical conduction in the heart muscle, causing it to beat more slowly, which is sometimes desirable.

A calcium channel blocker has been combined with a cholesterol-lowering medication. This medication is Caduet, which is a combination of amlodipine and atorvastatin.

DIURETICS ("Water Pills")

Diuretics are medications like Lasix (furosemide) and Hydrochlorothiazide (HCTZ) that lower the blood pressure by reducing blood volume and the body's salt content. Some have a direct relaxing effect on the blood vessels. They are usually added onto other blood pressure medications and are rarely used alone.

Many combinations exist, such as Diovan-HCT, Benicar-HCT, and Atacand-HCT. The combinations are useful because they reduce the number of tablets to be taken.

Patients taking these diuretics need to be under a doctor's supervision to make certain that dehydration is avoided and that the potassium level remains appropriate. Sometimes physicians prescribe additional potassium tablets or suggest their patients increase potassium consumption through foods such as chicken, lamb, bananas, and honeydew melon. Diabetics, of course, must be careful not to eat too many fruits because of the carbohydrate content.

Consult with your doctor before adding — or stopping — any medication or dietary supplement.

Four more medications are used in special circumstances:
- Alpha-1 Blockers are used mainly to ease bladder outlet obstruction in men with enlarged prostate glands. Care must be taken when Alpha-1 Blockers are used in combination with other blood pressure medications in order to prevent the blood pressure from falling too low.
- Central Alpha Agonists (clonidine and methyldopa) reduce blood pressure by blocking the sympathetic nerves which cause arterial narrowing.
- Aldosterone Receptor Blockers (like eplerenone) lower blood pressure by preventing salt retention.
- Vasodilators (like hydralazine) relax the muscles in blood vessel walls.

ALDOSTERONE ANTAGONISTS

Aldosterone Antagonists block the action of aldosterone, which is one of the hormonal mechanisms causing high blood pressure. One such medication is Aldactone (spironolactone). Aldactazide is a combination of Aldactone and hydrochlorothiazide (HCTZ), which can be more effective for some patients than either drug alone.

RENIN INHIBITORS

Currently under study and awaiting FDA approval, there is a new medication to block renin, the enzyme that changes angiotensinogen into angiotensin I *(Fig 5)*.

10

TREATING INSULIN RESISTANCE IN THE METABOLIC SYNDROME

Insulin resistance is an important problem in both the metabolic syndrome and in diabetes. When cells in our bodies become insulin resistant, they cannot process glucose, fat or protein efficiently.

Insulin is made by the beta cells in the pancreas. It allows glucose to enter cells where it can be used for energy or converted into a storage form called glycogen.

Insulin also plays a major role in fat and protein metabolism. Fat and protein metabolism are therefore disturbed when insulin resistance is present.

With insulin resistance, glucose does not enter cells efficiently. In the metabolic syndrome, this causes blood sugar to rise slightly — but not as high as in diabetes. The beta cells in the pancreas begin to make more insulin, trying to overcome the resistance, and blood insulin levels become elevated, a condition known as hyperinsulinemia.

Eventually, after some years, the beta cells become fatigued. Then insulin production drops significantly and the blood sugar rises to diabetic levels. By the time diabetes occurs, it is estimated that over half of the beta cells have died.

The beta cells are also injured by being exposed to excessive fatty acids (lipotoxicity) and high sugar levels (glucotoxicity).

Although weight loss can decrease insulin resistance, it is extremely important that someone with insulin resistance be treated with medication.

■ Medications For Treating Insulin Resistance

One of the more important discoveries of modern medicine has been the development of drugs that specifically target insulin resistance. These drugs are called insulin-sensitizers.

Currently there are two categories: the TZDs and metformin. The most important are the Thia-zolidine-diones or TZDs for short. Two are currently available — Avandia (rosiglitazone) and Actos (pioglitazone).

It is beyond the scope of this book to describe the detailed chemistry of TZD action. Briefly, TZDs act within the nuclei of cells where they activate a factor called PPAR-Gamma (pronounced "pea-par gamma"). The letters stand for Peroxisome Proliferator Activated Receptor-Gamma. It is through PPAR-Gamma activation that TZDs are able to help insulin and change fat metabolism for the better.

The TZDs have been used extensively in the treatment of diabetes. They improve glucose utilization, thus decreasing blood glucose levels.

The TZDs have not been cleared officially for use in the metabolic syndrome, but more and more experts believe that they should be used *before* diabetes occurs.

In the metabolic syndrome, blood glucose levels are only slightly elevated due to insulin resistance, but it is extremely important to remember that insulin resistance produces major abnormalities in fat and protein metabolism in the metabolic syndrome as well as in diabetes.

Defective fat and protein metabolism cause vascular damage. By treating insulin resistance early in the metabolic syndrome, the onset of cardiovascular disease can be slowed down.

TZDs, when used in the metabolic syndrome, will not lower blood sugar to undesirable levels. Indeed, the main objective in using TZDs is to fight the insulin resistance of the metabolic syndrome.

Within cells, particularly the muscle cells which are the greatest consumers of glucose, there are two pathways for insulin action. The first pathway, known as the PI-3 Kinase pathway, allows glucose to enter cells to be used for energy and to be stored as glycogen for later use. With insulin resistance, this pathway is partially blocked, mainly by fatty acids.

When the blockage occurs, insulin acts through a different pathway known as the MAP-Kinase pathway. The MAP-Kinase pathway produces undesirable products that damage blood vessels, increase clotting, and encourage cell stickiness and the overgrowth of muscle inside the blood vessel walls.

The TZDs, by helping insulin to act using the PI-3 Kinase pathway, diminish insulin action via the MAP-Kinase pathway. By preventing insulin from following the harmful MAP-Kinase pathway, the TZDs protect the blood vessels and act as antagonists of clotting, cell stickiness and vascular muscle overgrowth. They are therefore very useful medications.

BENEFITS OF TZDs
There are at least ten reasons to use TZDs in treating the metabolic syndrome:

1. **TZDs delay the onset of type 2 diabetes** because they reduce insulin resistance and protect beta cells from working themselves to death. When beta cells are preserved, they can produce insulin more effectively, thereby avoiding the high blood sugar levels of diabetes.
    Some experts hold that "tired" beta cells produce an imperfect insulin called Pro-insulin, a "low-octane" variety of insulin which accounts to some extent for insulin inefficiency.

2. **TZDs lower blood insulin levels** by removing insulin resistance. A high insulin level in blood (hyperinsulinemia) has several bad outcomes, such as causing the kidneys to retain too much sodium leading to high blood pressure. Insulin can cause blood vessels to constrict, becoming narrower, and thus causing high blood pressure.

3. **TZDs hinder production of super oxides in vascular linings (the endothelium).** These super oxides interfere with the formation of nitric oxide, which is important for vascular health. Super oxides promote clotting, plaque formation and narrowing of blood vessels.

4. **TZDs change small, dense LDL-C particles** into larger and less harmful particles. They also improve the good HDL-C into more protective forms (HDL2 and HDL3).

5. **TZDs cause uncommitted stem cells to become storage-type fat cells** under the skin rather than the harmful fat cells located inside the abdomen. TZDs also cause the older fat cells in the abdomen to die.

6. **TZDs promote triglyceride storage in the newly-formed fat cells** thereby lowering blood triglyceride levels. They also remove fatty acids from circulation and from muscle cells where the fatty acids block the PI-3 Kinase pathway and interfere with efficient glucose utilization.

7. **TZDs reduce the formation of PAI-1** (pronounced "pie-one") a factor that interferes with clot-busting.

8. **TZDs reduce micro-albumin** excretion by the kidneys. Micro-albumin in the urine is a very strong predictor of heart and kidney disease.

9. **TZDs lower C-reactive protein** in the blood, a sign of vascular inflammation.

10. **TZDs slow the conversion of inactive cortisone into active cortisone** which causes fat to accumulate in the abdomen.

TZDs are available in combination with other medications: Avandamet is metformin plus Avandia. Avandaryl is Avandia plus Amaryl, and Duetact is pioglitazone plus glimiperide.

METFORMIN

Metformin slows down the glucose production by the liver. It also improves glucose utilization by cells, particularly the muscle cells, which qualifies it as an insulin sensitizer.

Metformin is prescribed for diabetics to lower their blood glucose, but it must be used cautiously, if at all, whenever there is liver or kidney disease.

Its role in metabolic syndrome has been clarified. In those patients who have moderately elevated blood sugars below the diabetic range, metformin can play an important role, particularly since **it promotes weight loss rather than weight gain.** Also, by keeping the blood sugar low, it can protect beta cells from becoming fatigued, thereby delaying the onset of diabetes.

Metformin also is used successfully in treating Polycystic Ovary Syndrome (POS) a pre-diabetic condition affecting females wherein the ovaries contain multiple cysts. POS causes obesity, infertility, irregular periods, excess facial hair, high blood pressure and even male-pattern baldness. Women with POS have arterial and heart disease at a young age.

Metformin helps women with POS lose weight, while it also reduces insulin resistance and androgen (male hormone) production, thereby regulating menstrual periods and decreasing male-type hairiness. In these women, metformin can also delay the onset of diabetes.

Metformin is marketed under various trade names such as Glucophage, Fortamet and Glumetza.

Metformin is available in combination with Avandia and called Avandamet. A combination of metformin and glyburide is marketed as Glucovance. Another medication, called ACTOplus met, combines Actos (pioglitazone) and metformin.

11

ADDITIONAL MEDICATIONS AND NEW TREATMENTS FOR METABOLIC SYNDROME

The following medications are also important in managing the metabolic syndrome.

■ Medications to Prevent Blood Clots

Patients with metabolic syndrome and diabetes are more likely to develop blood clots. To help prevent clotting, there are several approaches:

- Aspirin is usually prescribed in a daily dose of 81 mg, often called "baby aspirin."
- Other anti-clotting medications like Coumadin, (warfarin) and Plavix (clopidogrel) may be used to prevent clotting in special circumstances.
- The TZDs are used to promote clot-busting.
- Omega-3 fatty acids also prevent clotting.

■ Medications for Weight Loss

Appetite suppressants already available include Adipex-P, Ionamin (phentermine); Didrex (benzphetamine); Bontril PDM (phendimetrazine); and Meridia (sibutramine). They can be very helpful to start and maintain a weight-loss program, but long-term use is not recommended because they sometimes can raise blood pressure and increase nervousness, among other side-effects.

Medications may also be used to prevent complete digestion of fats and carbohydrates. Xenical (orlistat) blocks complete digestion of fats and Precose (acarbose) and Glyset (miglitol) block carbohydrate digestion. Although these medications can be helpful in a weight-loss plan, they can produce flatulence, diarrhea and abdominal discomfort.

As with other prescription drugs, these should be used under a doctor's supervision.

Many new medications are being developed to assist in weight loss. One, known as rimonabant, reduces the appetite — especially food cravings which can lead to unhealthy and unwise food choices. This drug is currently undergoing FDA approval.

■ New Medications to Lower Blood Sugar and Promote Weight Loss

Byetta (exenatide) and Symlin (pramlintide) have recently become available for treating diabetes. These prescription drugs are given by injection and may be used in conjunction with insulin and oral agents in diabetes.

> Byetta was developed after scientists studied the Gila monster (pronounced "He•lah") and its unusual eating habits. The Gila monster is a large, poisonous, prehistoric-looking lizard covered with bead-like scales in alternating rings of black and orange. It lives in the Southwestern desert and eats very little, feeding infrequently in the spring on bird eggs and small mammals, storing the food for hibernation during the winter.

The Gila monster produces an incretin hormone, first identified in the saliva of the lizard, which ensures slow stomach emptying and causes a diminished appetite.

This hormone has been isolated, and the chemical structure replicated. Now, the FDA-approved injectable drug, Byetta, regulates glucose and stimulates insulin production. It also slows the emptying of the stomach and suppresses hunger, encouraging weight loss.

> **Precaution:** Byetta is not a substitute for insulin. It is not for use by type 1 diabetics, or patients with end-stage renal disease or severe gastrointestinal problems. It should *always* be used with proper medical supervision.

Recently it was discovered that humans make hormones in the intestine that are similar to Byetta. These hormones slow down stomach emptying and dispel hunger. However, these hormones are inactivated too quickly by an enzyme called dipeptidyl peptidase-4.

A new medication, Januvia (sitagliptin), is now available to block dipeptidyl peptidase-4 and prolong the action of naturally occurring incretins, thus controlling blood sugar and promoting weight loss.

As always, consult with your doctor before starting or stopping any medication. Be especially careful of adding any over-the-counter or health-store supplements to your prescribed medications without consulting your doctor.

Symlin is another drug recently introduced to treat diabetes, including type 1 diabetes. It is a synthetic form of a hormone called amylin, secreted by the pancreatic beta cells. It slows stomach emptying, creates a feeling of fullness and therefore decreases food intake. It interferes with a hormone called glucagon, also made by the pancreas, which raises blood sugar levels.

It is interesting to note that glucagon, by injection, has been used for many years by emergency medical personnel to correct low blood sugar reactions to insulin.

These new agents will very likely find a place in treating obesity in the metabolic syndrome.

■ The Link Between Metabolic Syndrome and Type 2 Diabetes: Understanding the Connection

Many people do not find out they are diabetic until they have their first heart attack. It does not have to be this way. Ordinary blood tests can yield information telling a physician if someone is predisposed to type 2 diabetes 10 — 15 — even 20 years before the actual onset of symptoms.

If you took the self-test in the first chapter, and found you have three of the five pre-diabetic markers, you need to be tested. If the results are negative and you do not yet have the metabolic syndrome or type 2 diabetes, you need to be very vigilant. Your doctor may prescribe medications and urge you either to start — or increase — your exercise program. You will also probably need to be much more careful of your food choices and eating patterns.

However, if the results are positive and you do have the metabolic syndrome or even type 2 diabetes, your doctor will most likely take a more aggressive approach. Not only will your diet and exercise plan be scrutinized and suggestions made for improvement, but your doctor will nearly always prescribe medications for blood pressure control and cholesterol improvement.

Early diagnosis and aggressive treatment of the metabolic syndrome incorporating diet, exercise and appropriate medications will delay the onset of diabetes and can sometimes prevent it altogether.

More importantly, such treatment will prevent, slow down, or even reverse the arterial damage that precedes diabetes by many years.

The transition from metabolic syndrome to type 2 diabetes can be uneventful with gradual onset of fatigue, thirst, frequent urination and sexual difficulties. Painful neuritis, vision loss and disorders of kidney and bowel function signal diabetes.

When elevated sugar (blood glucose) arrives, the glucose combines with proteins to form glycated end products which further damage blood vessels.

This elevated blood sugar typical of diabetes causes *microvascular* (small blood vessel) damage in eyes, the kidneys, and nerves, and it adds to the *macrovascular* (large blood vessel) damage of the metabolic syndrome. This is the damage that results in heart attacks and strokes due to high blood pressure and cholesterol abnormalities.

If you are a diabetic, you will need to enlist the help of family and friends. Help educate them about your disease so they can become part of your support network. And, of course, it is quite possible that they, too, may be at risk for diabetes and should be tested.

Diabetes requires the need for frequent glucose monitoring and using medications like glyburide, glipizide and insulin to lower blood glucose. Diabetics need ongoing medical supervision.

In addition to the symptoms already mentioned, people with diabetes experience other problems. Some include economic problems, such as having to take more sick days, which impacts both the employee and the employer. There is an accompanying loss of income and certain economic stress. Diabetes brings about an increased inability to work and earn a living. Very often, diabetes can affect the ease of obtaining health and life insurance. Additionally, rates are often higher than those paid by non-diabetics.

Other problems involve family issues, such as the enormous disruption of family life when the need arises to care for a disabled, blind, or paralyzed relative. Sometimes these are solely emotional problems, and other times they are bound up with economic issues.

And, of course, the diabetic faces personal health issues. Diabetic women may face infertility as well as a higher rate of miscarriages than non-diabetic women. Diabetic mothers face difficult pregnancies and difficult births due to large babies.

Other diabetic health issues facing both men and women include more frequent hospitalizations, slower recovery from illness and surgery, and susceptibility to infection, very often including tuberculosis.

Depression and anxiety are more prevalent among diabetics, and these mental states may be linked to family and economic issues as well, making for a very complicated health situation.

Additionally, a recent Japanese study suggests there may be a link between diabetes and certain types of cancer. Insulin can act as a stimulant, causing some cells to grow excessively.

None of this is good news. However, the positive note is that type 2 diabetes can be prevented. The diagnostic tests are widely available; contributing factors are easily identified; and the disease is very much preventable. In the early stages, type 2 diabetes is, to some extent, also reversible.

A Tale of Two Sisters

The two Hispanic sisters came from a long line of type 2 diabetics. By the time they reached their mid-40's, their father had already died from the complications of diabetes. The sisters avoided doctors. Both overweight, they did not want to weigh in or listen to a "diet-and-exercise-speech." They never had blood work done, nor did they test their blood sugar or blood pressure. They both claimed to feel fine and continued to eat fatty and starchy foods and sweets.

Always close, the sisters spent a lot of time together. By the time she was 47, the younger sister started complaining of tiredness and fatigue. As the months wore on, she lost a little weight, though she claimed she wasn't dieting. By Thanksgiving, she dragged herself to the family gathering but said she felt awful and probably had the flu. The family agreed that she looked sick. Some who hadn't seen her for a while were surprised at her weakness and pallor.

By Christmas, she felt even worse and was calling in to work, saying she was sick. By then, she had developed lower back pain, and thinking she might have a bladder infection, she medicated herself by drinking a lot of cranberry juice. The back pain worsened.

She told her sister that the flu had left her with "cotton mouth." She drank lots of water, but her thirst was never satisfied. And she said she was tired of getting up all night to go to the bathroom. The back pain had worsened.

She didn't show up to the family gathering on Christmas. She was just too sick. A few days later, her sister began thinking it wasn't the flu after all, and she started listing the symptoms.

"I think you have diabetes. You need to see a doctor."

The younger sister agreed, wondering why they hadn't figured this out sooner.

Later that same night, she felt worse. She could hardly even walk. At about 5 a.m. she called her family gasping, "I can't breathe. I need help!"

Seeing her, it was obvious she was in a desperate condition. Within minutes, she was rescued by ambulance and raced to the hospital. She had suffered a serious heart attack.

An undiagnosed diabetic, the ravages of the disease had been eating away at her for years. The runaway diabetes not only caused the heart attack, but she was suffering from ketoacidosis, a serious condition. And, furthermore, an abscess was discovered on her spine, a complication of the disease.

Diabetes had a stranglehold on her.

It took nearly a month in the ICU to ensure her survival. Extraordinary measures were taken to save her life. Ultimately, she received triple by-pass and heart-valve replacement surgery. Her recovery was slow.

From her hospital bed, she begged her sister to go and get tested for diabetes.

And she did. Her sister's blood work showed she was headed in the same direction — high trigylcerides and low HDL. She had the metabolic syndrome and was insulin-resistant — a classic pre-diabetic.

Her doctor explained how she could prevent diabetes, and he put her on a statin to improve her cholesterol and another medication to help her pancreas produce more efficient insulin. Within a month, her blood work showed dramatic improvement.

With the proper medications, a low carbohydrate diet, she now maintains normal blood sugar, good health, and is preventing type 2 diabetes.

The two sisters now compare their blood sugar results and both watch what they eat. One is diabetic, and the other is pre-diabetic and trying diligently to prevent it.

This story illustrates the importance of knowing your family history. However, even if there is diabetes in your family, those "bad" genes only set the stage for developing diabetes. What happens on that stage is under your control, but you must act now! Make wiser food choices, start moving more, and get tested.

12

COMPLICATIONS OF DIABETES: WHY PREVENTING TYPE 2 DIABETES IS SO IMPORTANT

If the onset of diabetes is prevented or delayed, the complications of diabetes can be avoided. These complications cause enormous suffering in affected individuals and their families.

When families are suddenly faced with a blind person in the house, an amputee, a stroke victim confined to a wheelchair, or a relative who must be taken to a dialysis center three times a week, major family stresses are certain to arise. Adjustments and coping skills are often beyond the financial and psychological abilities of family members.

Diabetic Eye Diseases

Diabetes affects the retina. Small aneurysms (micro-aneurysms) and small hemorrhages are seen early. Later, white areas called "exudates" develop. These are sometimes called "cotton wool" spots. Then, new blood vessels grow into the retina, the optic disc and the iris, by a process called neo-vascularization. Hemorrhages and retinal detachment follow, leading to blindness. Massive hemorrhage and scar tissue can be removed by surgery known as "vitrectomy," which may restore some vision.

When diabetes is first diagnosed, it is important that an opthalmologist perform a complete baseline examination of the eyes. Thereafter, an eye exam should be performed annually, or more often, if indicated. Better still, a complete eye examination should be done when the metabolic syndrome is suspected.

> In the United States, diabetic retinal disease is the leading cause of blindness in persons between the ages of 20 and 65.

Vision can be preserved for a long time, and it is not wise to wait for visual disturbances to occur before having an eye examination. ACE inhibitors are particularly recommended to slow the progress of retinal disease in diabetics even if their blood pressure is normal.

Other eye problems caused by diabetes include cataracts, which are opacities of the lens. Neo-vascularization of the iris may block the free flow of fluid in the eyeball, resulting in raised pressure or glaucoma, another cause of eye pain and blindness.

The third, fourth and sixth cranial nerves, which feed into muscles of the eyeball, may be affected by diabetes, causing weakness and paralysis of the eyeball muscles and faulty movement of the eyeballs. This, in turn, will cause double vision and dizziness. Pain may accompany glaucoma and the cranial nerve problems, but is not a feature of early retinal disease.

Early diagnosis of retinal disease and neo-vascularization will allow effective treatment using lasers. The timing of these procedures is crucial. The leaking blood vessels can be sealed by laser photocoagulation, but laser treatment cannot restore lost vision.

■ Diabetic Heart Disease

Diabetes affects the coronary arteries, resulting in poor blood supply to the heart muscle and infarctions, or death of heart muscle.

Cardiomyopathy, heart muscle degeneration, and weakness also occur. In addition, there is a problem with the autonomic, or automatic, nerve control of the heart, causing rhythm problems.

The major cardiac complications resulting from diabetes follow:

- **Coronary artery disease (CAD)**

  CAD is the most frequent cause of death in diabetics. Not only is it more frequent in diabetics, but it is also much more extensive, affecting multiple, rather than single vessels, as well as the smaller capillaries. Pre-diabetics, persons with insulin resistance and the metabolic syndrome are equally at risk for CAD.

  The endothelial dysfunction underlying coronary artery disease and the higher tendency for clot formation and plaque rupture were described earlier.

> *It has been found that the presence of micro-albuminuria not only indicates diabetic kidney disease, but is also a powerful predictor of CAD, presumably because micro-albuminuria reflects endothelial damage.*

- **Cardiomyopathy**

  Malfunction of the heart muscle occurs aside from the presence of CAD. Heart failure — failure of the muscle to pump adequately or to relax adequately — is the result of this cardiomyopathy (heart muscle degeneration and weakness). The heart may be enlarged because the heart muscle fibers are weakened and stretched even before high blood pressure occurs.

• **Autonomic Dysfunction**

The autonomic nervous system controls unconscious body functions like heart rate, bowel function, and urination.

It is divided into two parts — sympathetic and parasympathetic. The sympathetic system raises heart rate and blood pressure and increases the rate of breathing, while the parasympathetic system has opposite effects.

In diabetes, both sympathetic and parasympathetic systems may be disturbed, leading to loss of the normal balance between them and resulting in such undesirable outcomes as rapid heart rate, narrowing of the coronary arteries and even sudden death.

> Patients with diabetes may not experience pain when they are having a heart attack. This is called a "silent myocardial infarction." Symptoms may be misleading and point to other diagnoses. These symptoms may include:
>
> - weakness
> - nausea
> - vomiting
> - confusion
> - shortness of breath
>
> These symptoms should not be ignored. If they occur, they should be evaluated by a physician immediately.

An electrocardiogram (EKG) might be helpful, especially if a previous one is available for comparison, illustrating again that a detailed medical exam is important when diabetes is first suspected. It should always include an EKG and detailed medical work-up.

- **Myocardial Infarction (Heart Attack)**
The outlook for diabetics after a heart attack is more serious than for non-diabetics, mainly because the associated car-diomyopathy tends to cause heart failure, but also because rhythm disturbances are more frequent and severe.

Diabetics benefit greatly from strict glucose control after a myocardial infarction. This allows them to recover more quickly and to avoid fatal complications.

Most patients will receive intravenous fluids after a heart attack, fluids which often contain glucose. Not only will the patient's ability to eat vary from one day to the next, but cer-tain tests may require an empty stomach and the patient will again receive intravenous fluids instead of being allowed food. Therefore, the blood sugar levels should be monitored very closely (every 2 or 3 hours) and should be controlled by intravenous insulin.

It is quite inadequate to base insulin doses on pre-meal testing of blood sugars and to regard blood sugars of 200 as acceptable.

The goal should be to maintain the blood sugar below 140/mg dl at all times while hospitalized.

After a heart attack, every diabetic patient should be main-tained on aspirin, a beta blocker and an ACE inhibitor to reduce the likelihood of further heart attacks. The dose of aspirin should probably be 325 mg per day, the usual tablet size, rather than the smaller 81 mg dose recommended for non-diabetics.

Because of the need for very strict glucose control, families of hospitalized patients should turn a deaf ear to a patient's request for outside foods and forbidden treats. Visitors who wish to bring gifts would be well advised to bring magazines, books, plants or flowers instead of food, cookies, or boxes of chocolates and candy.

From time to time when making hospital rounds, I have been surprised and appalled to see a patient's extremely high blood sugar record, only to be told later by family members that they had sneaked my patient a cheeseburger, fries and a large soda or milk shake "to make them feel better" or because they "felt so sorry for them for being in the hospital." Such ill-advised behavior interferes with patient care and may actually impede recovery.

Vascular and heart disease account for 80% of the deaths in diabetes. The risk of a heart attack or stroke is 2 to 4 times higher in a diabetic than a non-diabetic.

Diabetic Gastro-Intestinal Difficulties

The stomach and bowel, being under automatic or autonomic nerve control can, like the heart, suffer from imbalance between the sympathetic and parasympathetic systems. The imbalance can lead either to slow emptying of the stomach, called gastric stasis, or to rapid transit of food through the bowel resulting in diarrhea, incontinence, poor absorption of nutrition, colon spasm, and constipation.

Diabetics also have bio-chemical problems in the gastro-intestinal tract which contribute to abnormal functions, such as diarrhea, constipation, indigestion, and poor absorption of vitamins and minerals.

Diabetics often suffer from swallowing difficulties (dysphagia), nausea, vomiting, indigestion and diarrhea. Diminished anal sensation and sphincter tone may contribute to incontinence.

If gastro-intestinal symptoms are severe, or not relieved by simple measures, the patient should request a referral to a gastro-enterologist, particularly when abdominal pain is a prominent symptom. The symptoms may point toward significant impairment of the blood supply to the intestine (mesenteric ischemia) or to gallstones.

Detailed evaluation of gastro-intestinal function by gastroscopy, colonoscopy, stool sample and other analyses for poor absorption and measurements of intestinal transit should be performed by an experienced gastro-enterologist.

Medications are available now either to slow or speed up intestinal motility, gastric emptying and acid production. There are also medications to manage diarrhea, constipation, malabsorption and bacterial overgrowth. These medications require the expertise of physicians well-versed in their use.

■ Diabetic Kidney Disease

Kidney disease in diabetes affects the filtering blood vessels and the tubules collecting the filtrate. The changes in the blood vessels, like those elsewhere in the body, result from Advanced Glycemic End-products (AGEs) and endothelial inflammation brought about by insulin resistance, lipoprotein abnormalities and hypertension. These changes in the blood vessels occur also in the pre-diabetic metabolic syndrome.

Micro-albuminuria, defined as albumin (protein) excretion between 30 to 300 mg per day, appears first. This is followed by increased protein in the urine, hypertension and impaired renal function manifested by reduced filtration and accumulation of urea and creatinine in the blood. Finally, end-stage renal disease (ESRD) supervenes, requiring dialysis for survival.

> End Stage Renal Disease (ESRD) is a huge and costly public health problem. At the end of 2000, there were more than 372,000 ESRD patients in the Medicare-funded dialysis program. In about 40% of these patients, diabetes was the cause of ESRD.

Usually, physicians rely on blood levels of urea nitrogen (BUN) and creatinine to indicate renal dysfunction. However, by the time creatinine has increased by relatively few points, one half or more of the kidneys' filtering ability already has been lost. Therefore, it is better to measure either Creatinine Clearance or Glomerular Filtration Rate (GFR).

The Glomerular Filtration Rate (GFR) is calculated from a formula called the Creatinine Clearance. The only measurement needed for the calculation is the serum creatinine:

Creatinine Clearance Formula

$$GFR = \frac{(140 - age) \times weight\ in\ kg}{72 \times Serum\ Creatinine} = ml/minute$$

(Normal is 91 to 130 ml/minute)

In females the top number is multiplied by 0.85 to give the GFR.

Calculation of the GFR is important because it reveals how the kidneys are working. The GFR helps guide the physician in treatment.

In the middle stage between micro-albuminuria and ESRD, so much albumin (protein) may be lost in the urine, that the blood albumin level drops. An important function of albumin is to draw water back into the circulation, called osmotic pressure. When albumin falls to low levels, water escapes from blood vessels into tissues, causing edema. An example of edema is swelling of the legs.

The combination of edema, heavy albuminuria and low serum albumin is known as "nephrotic syndrome." At this stage, red blood cells and their remnants, called "casts," may be found in the urine along with fat (lipiduria), and there is a notable increase in blood cholesterol.

Another form of diabetic kidney disease is renal tubular acidosis, characterized by elevated serum potassium and a mild rise in serum creatinine.

When renal insufficiency occurs, the serum creatinine is above 3.0/100 ml. At this stage, anemia is present due to a lack of a kidney hormone called "erythropoietin," which stimulates the bone marrow to make red cells. Calcium and phosphorous metabolism are also disturbed.

Finally the kidneys fail completely and uremia supervenes. Uremia means that waste products like creatinine, urea nitrogen and uric acid accumulate in the blood and cause the affected person to feel unwell. Anemia, weakness, low blood pressure on standing, muscle twitching, edema, heart failure and failure of appetite round out the picture. Untreated, the patient lapses into a uremic coma and dies.

Treatment of diabetic kidney disease relies on blood pressure control, close glucose control, and the administration of ACE inhibitors. Glucose and blood pressure control must be nearly perfect to slow the progress of kidney disease. Blood pressure control may require the administration of beta blockers, calcium channel blockers, ARBs and other agents in addition to ACE inhibitors.

> Good blood pressure and glucose control will slow the progression of both kidney disease and neuritis in diabetes. ACE inhibitors are particularly recommended to slow the progress of kidney disease in diabetics even if their blood pressure is normal.

■ Urinary Tract Infections

Diabetics are susceptible to urinary tract infections. They are exposed to multiple medications because of the complexities of diabetes and also because type 2 diabetics often fall into an older age group for whom anti-arthritic and other drugs potentially harmful to the kidneys are prescribed. It is the physician's obligation to detect urinary tract infections promptly and to use every care in choosing medications for patients with diabetic kidney disease.

The patient should maintain good hydration by drinking plenty of water. Self-medication with herbal remedies, folk remedies, and over-the-counter drugs should be avoided.

Suspected bladder infections should be reported promptly. The patient should be referred to a kidney specialist or nephrologist whenever diabetic kidney disease is present.

■ Diabetic Neuropathy

The earliest indications of diabetic nerve damage occur in the feet. The physician will detect loss of sensation for light touch, vibration, pinprick and cold, usually in both feet equally. The usual symptoms include:

- numbness
- tingling
- burning
- achiness
- shooting pains

Somewhat later, motor function (the ability to use muscles) becomes affected. Flexion and extension of the toes and at the ankles is affected. Eventually symptoms affect both legs. Next, the symptoms and signs may appear in the fingers, hands, forearms and even the trunk. This form of neuropathy is described as "symmetrical peripheral polyneuropathy."

Neuropathy may also be asymmetrical. It often affects one or more cranial nerves feeding the eye muscles. The most common form, "oculomotor paralysis," or third nerve paralysis is manifested by pain in or behind the eye, drooping of the upper lid, and outward deviation of the eye because of the unopposed action of the outer muscle innervated, or supplied, by the sixth nerve.

Asymmetrical neuropathy may also affect the chest and abdomen. Pain on one side, traveling from back to front in a narrow band along the course of a spinal nerve, can be quite severe and cause confusion with other chest and abdominal diseases. This presentation is like "shingles," except that the blisters of the shingles rash do not appear.

The treatment of diabetic neuropathy includes good control of glucose, hypertension and lipid abnormalities. The most troublesome aspect of neuropathy is the pain associated with it. Narcotic dependency can become a problem. Highly favored medications include anti-depressants, anti-epileptic drugs, and topical analgesics or surface anesthetics.

Referral to a neurologist is generally a good idea and should be requested.

■ Peripheral Vascular Disease

Peripheral Vascular Disease (PVD), meaning poor circulation in the legs, is associated with a high incidence of heart attacks and strokes. This poor circulation in the lower extremities fosters skin breakdown and infection, as well as ulceration. Healing is very slow due to poor blood supply. Skin grafting is often required. Infection is common and may require prolonged use of both local and systemic antibiotics.

A complete diabetic evaluation carefully assesses circulation in the legs and feet, noting:
• skin temperatures
• pulses
• skin discoloration (blueness, redness or paleness)
• pain in the calf muscles on walking (claudication)
• night pain relieved by letting the feet hang down
• absence of hair on the feet and toes

These symptoms are reliable indications of poor circulation and need to be addressed by your physician.

■ Diabetic Skin Problems

Skin problems around the lower legs and feet are dangerous, painful, disabling and expensive complications of diabetes.

Prevention is extremely important. It cannot be emphasized enough to arrange an early consultation with a podiatrist, even in the pre-diabetic stage.

The feet are subject to constant trauma from weight bearing coupled with improper footwear, causing pressure breakdown on the balls of the feet, over calluses and hammer toes, over bunions and around the nails.

Scrupulous hygiene with regular bathing in warm — not hot — soapy water followed by careful drying, especially between the toes, is crucial. Skincare lotions should be applied regularly. Footwear must be ample in size, allowing the free circulation of air. Wearing soft, clean, cotton socks will prevent rubbing and chafing and will also protect the lower legs from scrapes and bumps.

Necrobiosis Lipoidica Diabeticorum is a skin condition that usually occurs on the shins as shiny, yellowish plaques with darker edges. The skin may become very thin and ulcerated.

Granuloma Annulare presents ring-like lesions with depressed centers occuring near the joints.

Acanthosis Nigricans is a brown-to-blackish area occurring in the armpits, under the breasts, or along the sides and back of the neck. The skin ridges are velvety soft. It is common in obesity and diabetes, but may also point to an internal malignancy in non-diabetics.

Diabetic Dermopathy consists of small, reddish or brownish spots often seen on the shins. Biopsies have revealed small arteries almost completely closed by inflammation.

Thick, waxy skin often appears on the backs of the hands and fingers. Sometimes the skin looks "pebbly."

Scleredema is a similar lesion with thickening and stiffness of the skin in the nape of the neck and down the upper back and across the shoulders. Skin lesions are thought to be caused by an alteration in collagen in diabetics.

Blisters may appear quite suddenly on the feet and hands without any known precipitating cause.

Xanthomas are small red, round areas that appear on the arms, legs and buttocks, when triglyceride blood levels rise suddenly. They change to an orange color and then to yellow. Biopsy reveals cells laden with lipids in the skin.

Yeast infections are more common in diabetics than non-diabetics. Rashes may appear in the groin, breast folds, armpits, and around the anus and vulva.

Referral to a dermatologist or to a wound care center may be required if good diabetic control and simple measures do not relieve any of the above skin problems associated with diabetes.

A Nursing Student Sees the Pain of Diabetic Wounds

As a nursing student, learning about diabetes in my textbooks and caring for patients with the disease were two totally different experiences for me. On one of my clinical rotations, it was my job to cleanse a diabetic ulcer. I didn't realize how severe a diabetic wound could be until then. It was a tough experience for me.

When I got acquainted with the patient, I realized how much pain she was in, but I knew her nurse had already given her adequate pain medication for the procedure. I just didn't want to cause her more pain. Then I took a deep breath and began the cleansing routine used for a diabetic ulcer.

Once I had carefully removed the old dressing, it was hard to believe what I was seeing. This huge fleshy wound smelled awful and had black areas where the tissue was already dead from lack of circulation. I felt bad knowing the wound would take a very long time to heal — if it could ever heal — and that was a terrible thought. I cleansed the wound with saline and gently repacked it.

I was reminded how grateful I am for my health and well being. If there were any way that this patient's suffering could have been lessened, that would have been my wish.

Kelly Hilcove
Scottsdale, AZ

■ Diabetic Sexual Dysfunction

Erectile dysfunction is often an early complaint in diabetic males. Both males and females may also experience loss of libido. Tiredness, weakness and depression contribute to these problems. Patients should discuss these conditions with their doctor.

■ Diabetic Psychological Problems

Depression and anxiety are common in diabetics, particularly when the disease manifests peculiar skin rashes, painful neuropathy, life-threatening heart disease and strokes, as well as kidney failure.

Often, patients know of family members who died relatively young of cardio-vascular complications, or who suffered blindness or multiple amputations. This increases their anxiety, and it needs to be addressed through positive reinforcement and frequent reminders of the benefits to be derived from good diabetic control.

Psychiatric and psychological intervention should receive high priority in diabetics who may manifest denial, depression and suicidal thoughts, particularly in an unsupportive family environment. Financial problems related to illness, medical costs, lack of insurance and unemployment are major factors affecting the psychological well-being of many diabetics.

■ Diabetic Central Nervous System Disorders

Diabetes plus hypertension increases the risk of silent strokes, called "silent cerebral infarcts." When older adults have both diabetes and hypertension, they are more likely to suffer silent strokes than if they have hypertension alone. In some studies, about 80% of patients with both hypertension and diabetes had evidence of at least one silent stroke.

■ Lesser-Known Markers of Type 2 Diabetes

- Gestational Diabetes (diabetes during pregnancy)

- Frozen Shoulder

- Carpal Tunnel Syndrome

- Stiff Hands (unable to assume "prayerlike" position)

- Dupuytren's Contracture (hardened, ropelike tissue, pulling the 4th and 5th fingers down)

- Tendinitis of hands and ankles (pain and stiffness of joints)

- Cataracts of the eyes

- Frequent Urinary Tract Infection (UTI) and vaginal yeast infections

- Susceptibility to skin infection (for example, boils and slow healing wounds)

- Susceptibility to colds, pneumonia, coughs

- Polycystic Ovary Syndrome (POS) (excess facial hair, few menstrual periods, sterility)

- Cholesterol gallstones

- Fatty infiltration of liver

- Some cancers (excess insulin behaves as a growth factor)

Diabetes Is Dead Serious

When someone hears that a friend or relative has cancer, they shudder, picturing the horrors of the disease. When the diagnosis is diabetes, they often react as if it is a little allergy to sugar. "No more hot fudge sundaes for you," they joke.

Diabetes should scare the hell out of people. It is a bigger killer than cancer. Often, even diabetics don't take it seriously enough. They don't understand that it is a potentially devastating cardiovascular disease.

I know. I watched the ravages of diabetes kill my husband.

It wasn't until his first heart attack that we discovered he had type 2 diabetes. We didn't understand that diabetes had caused the heart attack. We thought they were two separate conditions.

We didn't understand that high blood sugar meant that damage was being done in his arteries, throughout his entire vascular system. Maybe if high blood sugar had a different, more frightening name, he wouldn't have been so casual about it.

Diabetes became his nemesis. In spite of trying to manage his blood sugar, he suffered two more heart attacks, cardiac arrest, continual congestive heart failure. At our house, it was life on the edge. Our kids didn't need to watch scary movies.

Not only was his heart failing, his kidneys began to fail.

Diabetes is relentless.

Failing kidneys meant dialysis. Since his heart was so weak, we learned to perform peritoneal dialysis at home — hemo-dialysis was not an option for him. A surgical procedure gave him a tube in his abdomen, and that was used to do the dialysis procedure three-times-a-day, every day.

Life on the edge had reached a new level.

Unfortunately, dialysis can only eliminate half of the body's toxins and, for him, after two years it no longer worked. Even at five-times-a-day, dialysis couldn't save him — we couldn't save him. Uremic poisoning from the failed kidneys took his life. His vascular system had been destroyed by diabetes. Diabetes robbed him of his life and robbed us of a husband and a father.

I know the truth: diabetes is dead serious.

Patricia Bezunartea
Scottsdale, AZ

HOPE FOR THE FUTURE

The complications of diabetes, and the suffering caused by these complications, illustrate how important it is to prevent diabetes by diagnosing pre-diabetics and treating the disease aggressively and early.

The public needs to be reminded constantly that obesity, overeating, lack of exercise, high blood pressure, and cholesterol abnormalities predict disaster. The children of diabetic families should immediately be treated for metabolic syndrome and started on a program to prevent type 2 diabetes.

If one thinks of the individual suffering and pain, the disruption of family life and the economic impact of diabetes on individuals, families, communities and nations, every effort to prevent diabetes is worthwhile.

At all levels, we need to mount a vigorous campaign to prevent type 2 diabetes. We have the knowledge and the tools to prevent this horrible disease, and because we can prevent it, we must.

GLOSSARY

A1C **(Hemoglobin "A-one-C" or glycated hemoglobin):** A test which measures the percentage of red pigment in the red blood cells (hemoglobin) that is combined with glucose. Once combined with hemoglobin, glucose remains in the red cell for the life of that cell which averages 90 days. The A1C test reveals whether the blood sugar has been well controlled for the preceding 90 days. A normal reading is 6%.

Actos (pioglitazone): A TZD that improves insulin sensitivity.

Advanced cholesterol test: A blood test providing information about the amounts of VLDL, LDL, HDL and triglyceride in the blood, as well as particle size of both LDL and HDL. Small particles of HDL are less protective than larger particles. Small LDL particles are more harmful than larger ones.

Alpha-blockers: Drugs used to treat elevated blood pressure. They block alpha receptors in blood vessels, *not* alpha cells in the pancreas.

Alpha cells: Cells found in the pancreas. They produce glucagon, a hormone that increases blood sugar. Glucagon converts stored sugar (glycogen) in the liver and muscles into glucose.

Amaryl (glimiperide): An oral drug of the sulfonylurea class given once a day. It stimulates beta cells to produce insulin.

Amino acids: The building blocks of proteins. Protein in food is digested down to amino acids.

Amylin: A hormone produced by beta cells in the pancreas to slow stomach-emptying and oppose the glucose-elevating action of glucagon. Now available in synthetic form as Symlin (pramlintide), it is given by injection to both type 1 and type 2 diabetics to control blood sugars and promote weight loss.

Apoprotein: The protein in the outer coat of a lipid molecule, encasing triglyceride and cholesterol. It enables the lipid to become soluble and react with other chemicals.

Aspirin: A drug used to prevent heart and blood vessel disease and to diminish clot formation by reducing platelet stickiness. It is usually prescribed in a daily dose of 81mg, called "baby aspirin."

Atherosclerosis: A disease characterized by hardening, loss of elasticity and plaque formation in the arteries.

Avandia (rosiglitazone): A drug of the thia-zolidine-dione class (a TZD) which improves sensitivity to insulin.

Beta blockers: Drugs for lowering blood pressure by blocking beta nerve receptors in blood vessels (*not* beta cells).

Beta cells: Cells in the pancreas that produce insulin and amylin. Also written as β cells. In the metabolic syndrome (pre-diabetes), they work at top-speed to produce insulin to control the blood sugar. This over-work causes them to fatigue and die. With fewer beta cells, less and less insulin is produced. Then the body is less capable of storing and using the excess glucose in the blood stream.

Although gene therapy promises the development of "replacement" beta cells, unless lifestyle changes are made and appropriate medications prescribed, the cycle of fatigued and dying beta cells will continue.

Blood pressure: The pressure measured in the brachial artery of the arm in millimeters of mercury (mmHg). Normally, the systolic blood pressure (after the heart has contracted) is 120 to 130 mm, whereas the diastolic pressure (when the heart is relaxed) is 70 to 80 mmHg.

"Borderline" diabetes: An incorrect and dangerous description for someone who is already diabetic, but whose blood sugar levels are only moderately elevated. These individuals are as likely to suffer diabetic complications as those persons with more elevated blood sugar, because they have the cholesterol and blood pressure abnormalities that cause arterial and heart disease. "Borderline" diabetes is like "borderline" pregnancy: it does not exist.

Calcium channel blockers: Drugs used to control blood pressure. They do not interfere with blood or bone calcium.

Carbohydrates: Starches and sugars present in all foods except meats, poultry, fish and fat. They contribute greatly to the levels of blood glucose and triglycerides.

Carbohydrate counting: A good way to know how much carbohydrate is being eaten. For example, a slice of bread contains 15 grams of carbohydrate. By controlling the daily intake of carbohydrates, diabetics can lose weight and control their blood glucose levels.

Cholesterol: A substance manufactured by the liver from fatty acids and absorbed from food containing fat and cholesterol. Cholesterol is a component of lipid molecules, bile, cell membranes and hormones. The cholesterol measured by blood tests is part of the lipoproteins LDL, VLDL, IDL and HDL (see separate entries).

C-reactive protein (CRP): A blood test which points to inflammatory processes in the body, such as blood vessel inflammation. It may be elevated in dental and gum infections and diseases like arthritis. It can be a useful predictor of cardiovascular incidents.

Crestor (rosuvistatin): A statin drug for lowering cholesterol and raising the good cholesterol, HDL.

Diabeta and Glucotrol XL (glyburide and glipizide): Sulfonylurea drugs given orally to reduce blood sugar by stimulating the pancreas to make more insulin.

Diabetes mellitus: A disease in which blood glucose is elevated both in the fasting state and after meals, because the pancreatic beta cells make too little insulin. Although abnormalities in blood glucose are the distinguishing characteristics, diabetes is also a cardiovascular disease caused by the cholesterol abnormalities and high blood pressure which are usually present. In type 1 diabetes, there is a total failure of insulin production due to beta cell death usually early in life, whereas type 2 diabetes is more commonly a progressive failure of insulin production in adult life from increasing beta cell fatigue.

The term "diabetes mellitus" is derived from Greek and Latin origins which emphasize frequent urination (L. *diabetes,* a siphon and GR. *diabainein* to pass through) and the sweet, honey-flavored urine (L. *mel,* honey).

Diabetic dermopathy: An inclusive term for skin abnormalities in diabetic patients.

Diabetic diet: A food management program that features decreased calories, fewer but healthier servings of carbohydrates, reduced fat and reduced salt. It is designed primarily to achieve weight loss, lower cholesterol and triglycerides, control blood pressure and lower blood glucose levels. A similar diet is prescribed for patients with metabolic syndrome.

Diabetic nephropathy: Kidney disease caused by diabetes, often ending in kidney failure and the need for dialysis. End-stage renal disease (kidney disease) is abbreviated ESRD.

Diabetic neuropathy: A disease of the nerves, usually affecting the legs and causing pain, loss of sensation, burning and tingling. Sensory loss can lead to injury caused by ill-fitting shoes, for example. This in turn can cause ulceration and infection so severe that amputation is necessary. Neuropathic pain is extremely severe and can lead to drug dependence, depression and suicide.

Diabetic retinopathy: A disease of the small arteries in the retina of the eye causing blindness.

Dyslipidemia: An inclusive term for cholesterol and triglyceride abnormalities.

Endothelium: The inner lining of blood vessels and the site of inflammatory changes in the metabolic syndrome and diabetes. Normally a smooth, shiny, flexible lining, it becomes rough and sticky when diseased, permitting plaque and blood clots to form.

Fatty acids: The end products of fat digestion absorbed from the intestine and converted by the liver into triglycerides. Fatty acids are also released from fat in the abdomen and converted into triglycerides and cholesterol by the liver. The fatty acids contribute to insulin resistance.

Fibrates: Medications prescribed to lower cholesterol and triglycerides and to raise HDL. See Chapter 8, "Treating Cholesterol Abnormalities."

Geranylgeranylation: A process by which harmful protein byproducts are formed during the synthesis of cholesterol. These byproducts contribute significantly to vascular disease and can be blocked by statin drugs.

Gestational diabetes: A form of diabetes that may develop during pregnancy. It may go into remission after delivery, but it signifies a tendency toward diabetes.

Glucagon: A hormone produced by alpha cells in the pancreas. It acts the opposite of insulin and raises the blood sugar when necessary, such as when a meal is missed. It causes stored sugar in the muscles and liver to be released into the blood stream.

Glucose: A sugar which is derived from food carbohydrates. Blood glucose levels are elevated in the metabolic syndrome and in diabetes. The normal fasting level is 100 mg-dl. After a meal, blood sugar should not rise above 160 mg-dl. If it does, the person is probably diabetic.

Glucose intolerance: A feature of the metabolic syndrome, or pre-diabetes, in which glucose is handled poorly, resulting from a combination of beta cell fatigue and insulin resistance. Both fasting and after-meal glucose levels are high, but not at diabetic levels.

Glycated end products: Combinations of glucose with proteins which damage blood vessels.

Glycemic index: An indication of a carbohydrate's ability to raise blood sugar. With sugar itself at 100, other carbohydrates are compared to it.

Glycogen: The form in which sugar is stored in the liver and muscles.

High density lipoprotein (HDL): A desirable form of cholesterol that is usually too low in metabolic syndrome and diabetes. It is a major risk factor for heart and vascular disease. The HDL transports the harmful LDL (low density lipoprotein) away from blood vessels.

Hyperlipidemia: A condition characterized by elevation of the blood lipids which are lipoproteins containing cholesterol and triglycerides.

Hypertension: Elevated blood pressure.

Insulin: A hormone made by beta cells in the pancreas. It controls blood sugar by facilitating the use and storage of glucose by cells, particularly muscle cells.

Insulin resistance: A defect in diabetes and the metabolic syndrome whereby glucose is incompletely utilized and stored by cells, resulting in elevated blood sugars and glucose intolerance, as well as the formation of undesirable products (glycated end products) which damage blood vessels and cause high blood pressure.

Isoprenoid: A protein, harmful to blood vessels. The formation of isoprenoids is facilitated by the enzyme reductase, which also facilitates the formation of cholesterol. The statins block the action of the reductase.

Low density lipoprotein (LDL): A form of cholesterol harmful to blood vessels when oxidized, and particularly harmful when present as small particles.

Lipitor (atorvastatin): A statin drug used to lower cholesterol, particularly LDL.

Lipoprotein: Particles composed of triglycerides and cholesterol, surrounded by a protein coat, called the apoprotein. The protein makes the particles soluble in the blood and enables them to react with other chemicals. Statins decrease triglyceride and cholesterol levels and are therefore very useful medications.

Lipoproteins are classified according to their density: Very Low Density Lipoproteins (VLDL), Intermediate Density Lipoproteins (IDL), and Low Density Lipoproteins (LDL). VLDL particles are the chief carriers of triglycerides. When blood is centrifuged, the lighter, low density VLDL particles rise to the top of the vial, and the heavier, high density particles remain at the bottom.

Metabolic syndrome: Not a true syndrome, but a useful concept describing obese individuals with large waistlines, high blood pressure, abnormal cholesterol and triglyceride levels and resistance to insulin. They may become diabetic, particularly when there is a family history of diabetes. These individuals are susceptible to cardiovascular disease such as heart attacks, strokes and blocked arteries whether or not they became diabetic.

Those who argue against calling it a syndrome, point out correctly that each of its components—obesity, hypertension and dyslipedemia—requires separate diagnosis and treatment emphasis. Another manisfestation—insulin resistance—is a core defect which causes suboptimal use and control of blood glucose. Insulin resistance contributes to "hyperinsulinemia" which, in itself, promotes cardiovascular disease.

Neoglucogenesis: A process by which glucose is formed in the liver from non-carbohydrate sources. This process is slowed down by metformin, a drug used in treating diabetes and the metabolic syndrome to regulate blood sugar.

Niaspan: A slow-release form of niacin used mainly to raise HDL and lower triglycerides.

Non-HDL cholesterol: A convenient term for the sum of all the undesirable cholesterols—VLDL, IDL and LDL. See VLDL entry.

Norvasc (amlodipine): A blood pressure medication of the dihydropyrdine class of calcium channel blockers. It lowers blood pressure by dilating blood vessels and by inhibiting sympathetic nervous control of blood vessels.

Omacor: A highly purified form of omega-3 fatty acids.

Omega-3 fatty acids: Organic acids found naturally in fish, walnuts, canola and flaxseed oils and added to other foods, such as eggs. Omega-3 can reduce triglycerides and is thought to reduce inflammation in blood vessels.

Reductase: An enzyme necessary for cholesterol synthesis. It also assists in the formation of isoprenoids, proteins that harm the blood vessels.

Statins: Drugs that lower cholesterol and reduce vascular inflammation by blocking the action of an enzyme (reductase) necessary for cholesterol synthesis. Reductase facilitates the formation of cholesterol from HMGCoA (3-hydroxy-2 methylglutaryl co-enzyme A) and the formation of proteins called isoprenoids, harmful to blood vessels. Therefore, by opposing reductase action, the statins slow down both cholesterol and isoprenoid production (Fig 5).

Triglycerides: End products of fat digestion absorbed from the intestine and processed by the liver. Triglycerides are then incorporated into lipoproteins. The lipoproteins are composed of triglycerides, cholesterol and a protein coat (apoprotein). Triglyceride levels are elevated in pre-diabetes and in diabetes and contribute significantly to cardiovascular disease.

VLDL, IDL and LDL: Lipoprotein particles that vary in density, with the Very Low Density Lipoproteins (VLDL) containing more of the light, fluffy triglyceride than cholesterol; the Intermediate Density Lipoproteins (IDL) containing about equal amounts; and the Low Density Lipoproteins (LDL) containing much more cholesterol than triglyceride. After a blood sample is obtained, the vial is spun in a centrifuge to measure the proportions of particles. The light, VLDL particles float to the top, creating a creamy looking "cap." Statins and fibrates decrease cholesterol and triglyceride levels.

Zetia (ezetemibe): A drug which interferes with the absorption of cholesterol from food. It is often added to or given with a statin to achieve ideal cholesterol goals. This allows the use of lower doses of statins and fibrates to decrease side effects.

Zocor (simvistatin): A member of the statin family of drugs.

BIBLIOGRAPHY

Bell, D.S.H., J. McGill. "Carvedilol Versus Metoprolol in Diabetic Hypertensive Patients." *Card Rev.* 2005. 22(10):12–17.

Brancati, F.L., N. Wong, L.A. Mead, et al. "Body Weight Patterns from 20 to 49 Years of Age and Subsequent Risk for Diabetes Mellitus." The Johns Hopkins Precursors Study. *Arch Intern Med.* 1999. 159:957–963.

Brennan, B.M., M.E. Cooper, D. de Zeeuw, et al. for the Renal Study Investigators. "Effects of Losartan on Renal and Cardiovascular Outcomes in Patients with Type 2 Diabetes and Nephropathy." *N Engl J Med.* 2001. 345:861–869.

Buchanan, T.A., A.H. Xiang, R.K. Pedone, et al. "Preservation of Pancreatic Beta Cell Function and Prevention of Type 2 Diabetes by Pharmacological Treatment of Insulin Resistance in High Risk Hispanic Women." *Diabetes.* 2002. 51:2796–2803.

Cenuth, S., K.G. Alberti, P. Bennet, et al. "Follow-up Report on the Diagnosis of Diabetes Mellitus." *Diabetes Care.* 2003. 26(11):3160.

Chiasson, J., R.G. Jesse, R. Gomis, et al, for the STOP-NIDDM Trial Research Group. "Acarbose for Prevention of Type 2 Diabetes Mellitus: The STOP-NIDDM Randomised Trial." *Lancet.* 2002. 359:2072–2077.

Desprès, Jean-Pierre. "Visceral Adipose Tissue and Its Contribution to Global Cardiometabolic Risk." *Baylor College of Medicine Reports on Cardiometabolic Disorders*. 2006. 3(1):1–9.

Diabetes Atorvastatin Lipid Intervention (DALI) Study Group. "The Effect of Aggressive Versus Standard Lipid Lowering by Atorvastatin on Diabetic Dyslipidemia." *Diabetes Care*. 2001. 24:1335–1341.

Diabetes Control and Complications Trial (DCCT) and Epidemiology of Diabetes Interventions and Complications Research Group. "Intensive Diabetes Therapy and Carotid Intima-Media Thickness in Type 1 Diabetes Mellitus." *N Engl J Med*. 2003. 348:2294–2303.

Diabetes Prevention Program Research Group. "Costs Associated with the Primary Prevention of Type 2 Diabetes Mellitus in the Diabetes Prevention Program." *Diabetes Care*. 2003. 26:36–47.

____. "The Effect of Intensive Lifestyle Intervention and Metformin on the Incidence of Metabolic Syndrome among Participants in the Diabetes Prevention Program (DPP)." Presented at the 63rd Scientific Sessions of the American Diabetes Association. New Orleans, LA. June 13–17, 2003.

____. "The Impact of Lifestyle and Metformin Therapy on Cardiovascular Risk Factors in the Diabetes Prevention Program." *Diabetes*. 2003. (Suppl). 52:A169, Abstract, 723-P.

____. "Prevention of Type 2 Diabetes with Troglitazone in the Diabetes Prevention Program." Presented at the 63rd Scientific Sessions of the American Diabetes Association. New Orleans, LA. June 13–17, 2003.

____. "Reduction in the Incidence of Type 2 Diabetes with Lifestyle Intervention or Metformin." *N Engl J Med*. 2002. 346:393-403.

FARB, et al. "Coronary Plaque Erosion Without Rupture into a Lipid Core: A Frequent Cause of Coronary Thrombosis in Sudden Coronary Death. *Circulation*. 1996. 93:1354–1363.

Fonarow, G.C. "The Role of Neurohormonal Antagonists in the Management of Patients with Hypertension, Metabolic Syndrome and Diabetes." *Card Rev.* 2004. (Suppl). 21:4.

Ford, E.S., W. H. Giles, W.H. Dietz. "Prevalence of the Metabolic Syndrome among US Adults: Findings from the National Health and Nutrition Examination Survey (NHANES)." *JAMA.* 2002. 287:356–359.

Gaede, P., P. Vedel, N. Larsen, et al. "Multifactorial Intervention and Cardiovascular Disease in Patients with Type 2 Diabetes." *N Engl J Med.* 2003. 348:383–393.

Gaede, P., P. Vedel, H. Parving, et al. "Intensified Multifunctional Intervention in Patients with Type 2 Diabetes Mellitus and Microalbuminaria." *Lancet.* 1999. 353:617–622.

Galassi, A., K. Reynolds, J. He. "Metabolic Syndrome and Risk of Cardiovascular Disease: A Meta-Analysis." *Am J Med.* 2006. 119:812–819.

Ganda, O. "Diabetes and 'Prediabetes' in Cardiovascular Disease: An Underestimated Problem." *Card Rev.* 2005. 22(4):18–20.

Gerstein, H.C., S. Yusef, J. Bosch, et al. "Effect of Rosiglitazone on the Frequency of Diabetes in Patients with Impaired Glucose Tolerance or Impaired Fasting Glucose: A Randomised Controlled Trial." *Lancet.* 2006. 368:1096–1105.

Giugliano, D., R. Acampora, R. Marfella, et al. "Metabolic and Cardiovascular Effects of Carvedilol and Atenolol in Non-insulin-dependent Diabetes Mellitus and Hypertension, A Randomized Controlled Trial." *Ann Intern Med.* 1997. 126:955–959.

Goodpaster, B.H., D.E. Kelly, R.R. Wong, et al. "Effects of Weight Loss on Regional Fat Distribution and Insulin Sensitivity in Obesity." *Diabetes.* 1999. 48:839–847.

Haffner, S.M., A.S. Greenberg, W.M. Weston, et al. "The Effect of Rosiglitazone Treatment on Non-traditional Markers of Cardiovascular Disease in Patients with Type 2 Diabetes Mellitus." *Circulation*. 2002. 106:679–684.

Heart Outcomes Prevention Evaluation (HOPE) Investigators. "Effects of Ramipril on Cardiovascular and Microvascular Outcomes in People with Diabetes Mellitus." Results of the HOPE Study and the MICRO-HOPE Substudy. *Lancet*. 2000. 355:253–259.

Heymsfield, S.B., K.R. Segal, J. Hauptman, C.P. Lucas, M.N. Boldrin, A. Rissanen, J.P.H. Wilding, L. Sjöström. "Effects of Weight Loss with Orlistat on Glucose Tolerance and Progression to Type 2 Diabetes in Obese Adults." *Arch of Intern Med*. 2000. 160(5):1321–1326.

Ho, K.K.L., J.L. Pinsky, W.B. Kannel, et al. "The Epidemiology of Heart Failure; The Framingham Study." *J Am Coll Cardiol*. 1993. 22:6A–13A.

Jacob S., K. Reff, E.J. Henricksen. "Anti-hypertensive Therapy and Insulin Sensitivity: So We Have to Redefine the Role of Beta-Blocking Agents?" *Am J Hypertens*. 1998. 11:1258–1265.

Johnson, L.W., R.S. Weinstock. "The Metabolic Syndrome: Concepts and Controversy." *Mayo Clin Proc*. 2006. 81(12):1615–1620.

Lindlolin, L.H., H. Ibsen. K. Borch-Johnson, et al. "Risk of New-Onset Diabetes in the Losartan Intervention for Endpoint Reduction in Hypertension Study (LIFE)." The LIFE Study Group J. *Hypertense*. 2002. 20:1879–1886.

Miller, J.L. "Insulin Resistance Syndrome: Description, Pathogenesis, and Management." *Type 2 Diabetes Management*. 2003. 1:27–34.

Moore, L.L., A.J. Visioni, P.W. Wilson, et al. "Can Sustained Weight Loss in Overweight Individuals Reduce the Risk of Diabetes Mellitus?" *Epidemiology*. 2000. 11:269–273.

Must, A., J. Spandana, E.H. Cookley, et al. "The Disease Burden Associated with Overweight and Obesity." *JAMA*. 1999. 252:1523–1539.

Pyrala, K., T. Pederson, J. Kjekshies, et al. "Cholesterol Lowering with Simvistatin Improves Prognosis of Diabetic Patients with Coronary Heart Disease." A Subgroup Analysis of the Scandinavian Simvistatin Survival Trial (4S). *Diabetes Care*. 1998. 20:614–620.

Rakel, R.E., M.A. Weiss. "Diabetes Care: Are We Asking the Right Questions?" *Consultant*. 2007. 5:549.

Sattai, N., A. Gaw, O. Scherbakova, et al. "Metabolic Syndrome with and without C-Reactive Protein as a Predictor of Coronary Heart Disease and Diabetes in the West of Scotland Coronary Prevention Study (WOSCOPS)." *Circulation*. 2003. 108:414–419.

Schillaci, G., M. Pirro, G. Vaudo, F. Gemelli, G. Pucci, E. Mannarino. "The Metabolic Syndrome and Essential Hypertension." *Card Rev*. 2005. 22(6):32–35.

Setji, T.L., A.J. Brown. "Polycystic Ovary Syndrome: Diagnosis and Treatment." *Am J Med*. 2007. 120:128–132.

Sowers, J.R. "Effects of Statins on the Vasculature: Implications for Aggressive Lipid Management in the Cardiovascular Metabolic Syndrome." *Am J Cardiol*. 2003. (Suppl). 91:14B–22B.

Toto, R.D. "Management of Hypertensive Chronic Kidney Disease: Role of Calcium Channel Blockers." *JCH*. 2005. (Suppl). 1:V7-NO4.

Tuomilehto, J., J. Lindstrom, J.G. Eriksson, et al. "Prevention of Type 2 Diabetes Mellitus by Changes in Lifestyle Among Subjects with Impaired Glucose Tolerance." *N Engl J Med*. 2001. 344:1343–1350.

United Kingdom Prospective Diabetes Study Group. "Intensive Blood Glucose Control with Sulphonylureas or Insulin Compared with Conventional Treatment and Risk of Complications in Patients with Type 2 Diabetes." *Lancet*. 1998. 352:837–853.

____. "Tight Blood Pressure Control and Risk of Macrovascular Complications in Type 2 Diabetes: UKPDS 38." *BMJ*. 1998. 317:703–713.

Utzschneider, K., C. Carr, S. Barnsness., et al. "Weight Loss Is Associated with Improvement in Beta Cell Function in Older Subjects." Presented at the 63rd Scientific Sessions of the American Diabetes Association. New Orleans, LA. June 13–17, 2003.

Williams, K., A. Bertoldo, C. Corbelli, et al. "Weight Loss Induced Plasticity of Skeletal Muscle Glucose Transport and Phosphorylation in the Insulin Resistance of Obesity and Type 2 Diabetes." Presented at the 63rd Scientific Sessions of the American Diabetes Association. New Orleans, LA. June 13–17, 2003.

Wong, R.R., E. Vendetti, J.M. Jakicic, et al. "Lifestyle Intervention in Overweight Individuals with a Family History of Diabetes." *Diabetes Care*. 1998. 21:350–359.

Xiang, A.H., R.K. Peters, S.I. Kjos, et al. "Pharmacological Treatment of Insulin Resistance at Two Different Stages in the Evolution of Type 2 Diabetes: Impact on Glucose Tolerance and β-Cell Function." *J Clin Endocrinol Metab*. 2004. 89:2846–2851.

Xiang, A.H., R.K. Peters, S.I. Kjos, A. Marroquin, J. Goico, C. Ochoa, M. Kawakubo, T.A. Buchanan. "Effect of Pioglitazone on Pancreatic β-Cell Function and Diabetes Risk in Hispanic Women with Prior Gestational Diabetes." *Diabetes*. 2006. 55:517–522.

INDEX

ABOUT THE AUTHOR

"After more than 50 years of treating diabetics, it is my sincere hope that we can reach many people with the understanding of metabolic syndrome and this message of prevention so that they can live normal, healthy lives free from the pain, suffering and the sadness of diabetes."

Dr. Gabriel Hilkovitz

Gabriel Hilkovitz, M.B., B.Ch., received his medical education and postgraduate hospital training in South Africa, England and the United States. After graduation from the University of Witwatersrand in Johannesburg, SA, he completed internship and residency training in South African teaching hospitals.

Accepting a post as a medical officer in the gold mines, he taught rescue workers methods of responding to underground mining disasters. He was among the first to use cortisone successfully in treating nitrous fumes poisoning, caused by underground explosions.

Following a period of medical practice in rural South Africa, he traveled to London for postgraduate hospital training. His research in sickle cell disease resulted in a fellowship award at the Medical College of Virginia. There he joined the teaching faculty as an Associate Professor of Medicine. He served as Director of Emergency and Outpatient Services and Director of Internships, while also serving as the Assistant Dean of Medical Education.

Deciding to leave the academic world, he returned to private medical practice, relocating to New Hampshire. In 1980 he moved to Phoenix, Arizona, re-establishing a private medical practice in a warmer climate, more to his liking as a South African native.

He continues a close working relationship with the Arizona Heart Institute, where he specializes in internal medicine and diabetes treatment. He frequently is engaged for seminars and speaking presentations.

Dr. Hilkovitz is currently writing a companion book about treating type 2 diabetes.

NOTES

WE WANT TO HEAR FROM YOU!

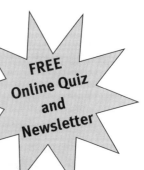

FREE
Online Quiz
and
Newsletter

- Do you know someone who has a story to share about their diabetes experience?

- Perhaps it's a way of coping with some of the problems associated with diabetes. Maybe it's a favorite recipe adapted to a healthier version. Is there a story connected with it?

- Maybe you would like to share a poignant—or humorous— insight into diabetes and the effects it has on diabetics, families and co-workers.

- Do you have ways of "Living Well" with diabetes? What healthy changes have you made in your life?

- How has diabetes affected your family? Your friends? Do you talk about it with them? Why or why not? What suggestions can you make for others?

- Give us your feedback about this book. What would you like to see in Dr. Hilkovitz's next book? Are there questions you'd like to ask him?

- **Type your narrative/recipe/suggestions/questions (200-word maximum) and send to:**

DIABETES NARRATIVE
BelVista Publishers, LLC
PO Box 2723
Scottsdale, AZ 85252-2723   USA

- Or, **email your submission (200-word maximum; no attachments)** to *www.narrative@belvistapublishers.com*

- Please include your name and mailing address; one submission per person. Not all material will be accepted, and submissions will be subject to editorial revision.

- **Please visit *www.info@belvistapublishers.com* for further infor-mation and to register for a free newsletter.**